P9-DID-103

Theories of Illness

GEORGE PETER MURDOCK

Theories of Illness

A World Survey

University of Pittsburgh Press

Published by the University of Pittsburgh Press, Pittsburgh, Pa., 15260
Copyright © 1980, University of Pittsburgh Press
Feffer and Simons, Inc., London
Manufactured in the United States of America

Library of Congress Cataloging in Publication Data

Murdock, George Peter, 1897–
  Theories of illness.

  Bibliography: p. 99
  Includes index.
    1. Medical anthropology. 2. Diseases—Causes and theories
of causation. 3. Medicine, Primitive.
  I. Title. [DNLM: 1. Cross-cultural comparison.
  2. Medicine, Primitive. 3. Philosophy, Medical.
  4. Anthropology. 5. Disease—Etiology. GN296 M974t]
  GN296.M87   362.1   80-5257
  ISBN 0-8229-3428-0

Chapter I, and portions of chapters II, III, and V originally appeared in
Ethnology, 17 (October 1978).

In remembrance of

John Philip Gillin

scholar, colleague, and cherished friend

Contents

Foreword

A new book by the distinguished anthropologist Professor George Peter Murdock is always a significant event, not only for colleagues in his own field but also for scholars in related fields. He brings to bear much more than conventional scholarship, for he is a strong individualist who shows us a novel methodology and numerous unexpected insights. He has been called the totemic ancestor of cross-cultural research because of his founding of the Human Relations Area Files and his lifetime involvement in comparative studies.

Medical historians, public health workers, and psychiatrists, as well as anthropologists, other social scientists, and interested laymen, have long been impressed by the value of comparative research. Such major interests as family relations, sexual practices, ecology and epidemiology, emotions and taboos, and the relationships between healers and patients justify the emerging specialty field of medical anthropology. *Theories of Illness* establishes a new landmark in comparative studies. Utilizing concepts from modern medicine and anthropological theory, Professor Murdock distinguishes the natural causes of illness from theories of supernatural causation. He subdivides the latter into theories of illness that are related to aggression (witchcraft, sorcery, and spirit aggression) and those which are related to guilt and a sense of sin (taboo violation and mystical retribution). Obviously, these relate to man's most basic beliefs as revealed in early religions. They also occur in some current belief systems as well as in the apparently spontaneous associations of persons who become seriously sick today without being aware of ancient customs. Readers of current books on newer concepts of living with pain, controlling fear and anger, and learning how to cope in the family with death and dying will recognize the relevance of this study.

To me the sheer magnitude of Professor Murdock's worldwide coverage is most impressive. He draws his data from 139 primitive, historical, and contemporary societies, selected as a "stratified sample" of the world's best-documented cultures on the model of those employed in the leading public-opinion polls. This number is far more than most of us can hope to visit or even read about.

It is not easy for me, not an expert in this field, to stress enough the vital importance of broadly based cross-cultural studies on theories of disease as related to aggression, magic, and mystical retribution. They are of great assistance in enabling us to avoid parochial, monothematic hypotheses. The regional differences found by the author serve to warn us of the possibilities of personal biases that may lie outside of our conscious awarenss of racial, ethnic, and religious differences.

The elucidation of the various facets of aggression in Chapters IX and X is highly valuable to many of us. It is surely one of the most ubiquitous and fascinating topics that has captured the attention of behavioral scientists as well as laymen. Its relations to manifold aspects of human conduct institutionalized in laws, rituals, codes of ethics, and religions continue to be a mystery in their spectacular variety. Not least in importance is Professor Murdock's observation that man everywhere has found ways to project his own aggressions outward to the supernatural beings he has created. It will not surprise modern readers that aggression is found to be a major motivation in supernatural theories of illness. Writings by serious investigators in the behavioral sciences, including those about psychophysiological relations, provide increasingly impressive evidence that it provides, for example, a partial basis for the formation of some types of cardiac and hypertensive disease. Of course, there is a large anecdotal and an increasing epidemiologic literature with suggestive if not entirely convincing data correlating strong emotions other than aggression, such as fear, frustration, guilt, helplessness, hopelessness, and depression, with most body systems. Interestingly enough, many early societies even recognized emotional tension or stress as a component of their theories of causation.

It is a matter of regret that technical difficulties prevented this study from covering those theories and practices in the gray zone between illnesses of natural and supernatural causation which are currently familiar to us as acupuncture, hypnosis, faith healing, and chiropractic and are sometimes associated with cults. Theories of illness in this gray zone, often ostensibly based upon modern molecular medicine, actually employ a relatively small number of basic assumptions found among the natural and supernatural theories of illness described in this book. As in earlier cultures, these techniques of the gray zone contain elements of validated empirical knowledge such as we now recognize in the phenomena of hypnosis, placebo effect, and neurotransmitters. We tend to assimilate them with such mechanisms as aggression, projection, and anxiety.

Not so incidentally, the consideration in Chapter XII of the desirability of enlightened sexual mores in our own society will probably be of more than casual interest to many readers. The surprising positive correlation of lax rather than strict early sex behavior with mystical retribution theories should be a source of major discussion and further investigation. All of us who have hoped that relaxed early sex socialization would result in greater freedom from internal conflict, including anxiety and guilt, may well want to reexamine our data and investigative methods.

Finally, for readers with both a sense of history and a sense of humor, this study provides confirmation for what is perhaps the first behavioral science hypothesis in history, namely, that advanced by Herodotus (ca. 484–425 B.C.) who suggested that people living in warmer climates are more sexually active and less inhibited than those in colder climes. Behavioral scientists can now investigate this aspect of our current period of affluence as a factor in the culture for growth we provide for our young.

—Henry W. Brosin, M.D.

Preface

To my family physician—and presumably to most readers—medicine is viewed as applied science, or more specifically as applied human biology. But to Johnny Quinn, the highly respected shaman who served as my principal informant among the Tenino Indians of Oregon, medicine was regarded quite differently—not as science in any sense but as applied religion. Most of the world's inhabitants including not a few members of our own society, for example, those who prefer prayer to penicillin, find themselves in much closer agreement with the medicine man than with the man of medicine.

This paradox of the contrast and overlap between medicine and religion has long fascinated me and, indeed, was among the attractions which first drew me into anthropology. My decision to investigate the theories by which man has sought to explain illness stems more from scientific curiosity than from any particular identification with the emerging field of medical anthropology. The exploratory character of this book has led to a number of serendipitous discoveries, which have contributed to its somewhat unorthodox order of presentation. It begins with a typology of the theories of illness encountered in a world survey, continues with an exposition of my theoretical orientation and methodology, then analyzes the geographical distribution of the major supernatural concepts of illness, and finally attempts to account scientifically for their occurrence, incidence, and perpetuation. I have also permitted myself occasionally to interject materials that seem pertinent and illuminating on subjects other than medicine and religion, most notably on language, aggression, sin, and sex.

This study was undertaken as part of a program of comparative research initiated at the University of Pittsburgh in 1969 with support from the National Science Foundation. The Cross-Cultural Cumulative Coding Center, as the program was called, produced a series of comparative studies under the direction of Herbert Barry III, Arthur Tuden, and me with the assistance of a staff of experienced coders. All applied comparable coding methods to a standard sample of the world's most fully described cultures, so that the results of each are capable of intercorrelation with those of the others.

For assistance in the preparation of this book, I am particularly grateful to the dedicated and meticulous coders who assessed the source materials: Edith Lauer, Catherine Marshall, Caterina Provost, and especially Suzanne Frayser (formerly Wilson) and Violetta Frederick. Professional colleagues who provided crucial information on societies they themselves have studied include Harold C. Conklin, Carleton S. Coon, Ward H. Goodenough, June Helm, and Samuel N. Kramer. Jean Adelman and Alice Schlegel rendered valuable library assistance, and Robert D. Murdock provided criticism and material help far beyond normal expectations in a son. Without the steadfast encouragement and the sophisticated technical advice of Douglas R. White, this book could not have been written. His planning and preparation of the statistical tables are particularly appreciated.

It also seems appropriate to mention with gratitude the behavioral scientists who, over the years, have exerted the most profound influence on my intellectual development. Albert G. Keller stimulated my lifelong interest in ethnography and instilled in me a deep respect for science and its methods. Edward Sapir introduced me to the fascinating field of linguistics and sponsored my initial exposure to field research—among the Haida Indians of British Columbia in 1932. John Dollard, Clark Hull, Mark A. May, and Neal E. Miller, as a result of interdisciplinary cooperation at the Institute of Human Relations, brought me to a realization of the basic role of behavioral psychology in the scientific study of man. Among anthropologists, John Gillin, A. I. Hallowell, Clyde Kluckhohn, Ralph Linton, and John Whiting are those with whom I have felt the closest comradeship in the common effort to convert our subject from a pleasurable antiquarian hobby to an eclectic scientific enterprise closely intermeshed with psychology and sociology.

Readers who agree with the approach and substance of this book may also be interested in the Society for Cross-Cultural Research, the organization before which I presented my first draft. Its offices rotate among anthropologists, psychologists, and sociologists, and its meetings provide a forum for lively and rewarding interdisciplinary interaction. Inquiries concerning membership or attendance at its February annual meetings may be addressed to the Society for Cross-Cultural Research, c/o Department of Anthropology, University of Pittsburgh, Pittsburgh, Pennsylvania 15260.

Theories of Illness

I

Primitive Medicine

Anthropological attention was first drawn to the significance of theories of illness in a pioneering paper by Forrest E. Clements (1932). It clearly demonstrated that the explanations of illness current among most of the peoples of the world have little in common with those recognized by modern medical science and relate much more closely to the ideology of primitive religion. Indeed, such scholars as Edward B. Tylor (1871) have suggested that religion itself is derived from them. This view will receive ample corroboration in this volume and, indeed, may be said to run through its pages like a leitmotif.

However, there exists a genuine danger that the reader who accepts it prematurely may form a seriously erroneous conception of primitive medicine and overlook its substantial component of sound pragmatic knowledge. In every human society countless generations have faced their health problems, like their technological problems, by trial-and-error behavior, during the course of which maladaptive responses have gradually given way to better adjustments in the normal cumulative process which we know as cultural evolution. To avoid misunderstanding in future chapters, it seems advisable to underline this point by citing examples of genuine medical achievements in several of the societies we shall consider, as reported in an earlier publication (Murdock 1934).

• Nama Hottentot (#1): "Other ailments are recognized to have natural causes and are treated by rational or pseudo-rational methods such as purgatives and emetics, herbal decoctions, dung poultices, and

3

applications of skin from a living animal. Broken limbs are set in splints. For localized pains the universal treatment is bleeding— either by opening a vein with the aid of a ligature or by cutting the skin and applying suction with a horn cup. A person bitten by a snake either applies to the wound a poultice made from the crushed body of the snake that bit him, or makes cuts around the wound and draws blood by cupping, or he calls in a special 'snake doctor.' The latter is a man who has immunized himself by swallowing or injecting into his skin various snake venoms in minute but gradually increasing doses, and who can transfer his immunity by rubbing sweat into incisions in his patient's skin" (p. 500).

• Ganda (#12): "Having learned the cause of the complaint, the medicine man may prescribe massage, sweat baths, cupping with a horn, blistering with a hot iron, or the internal or external use of various herbal remedies. The native practitioners are also adept at setting broken limbs in splints, and they have even been known to cure men partially disemboweled from spear wounds by washing the protruding intestines, forcing them gently back into the abdomen, and keeping them in place with a gourd" (p. 542).

• Samoans (#106): "The sick are invariably treated with the greatest consideration. The physicians who minister to them are often old women, each with her secret lore which she imparts only to her chosen successor, but there are also male shamans or medicine men. The therapeutic methods employed include emetics, ointments, massage, bleeding, and lancing. Cuts are bathed with salt water and bandaged with leaves. Fractured bones are set with considerable skill" (pp. 76–77).

• Aztec (#153): "The treatment of disease was a function of a special class of physicians or medicine men, who, says an ancient chronicler, 'were so far better than those in Europe that they did not protract the cure, in order to increase the pay.' These practitioners set fractured bones, sewed wounds with hair, prescribed bloodletting and sweat baths, and applied their knowledge of herbs in the preparation of various infusions, purgatives, emetics, and ointments" (p. 386).

• Inca (#171): "Therapeutic practices such as massage, bleeding, and the use of purgatives were primarily exorcistic in purpose, though more rational motives doubtless underlay bonesetting and the use of poultices and salves for sprains and wounds. . . . The *amautas* practiced trepanation of the skull for fractures from club blows and probably also for less adequate reasons. They scraped the surface of the bone with a stone knife, incised a square, circular, or irregular segment, forcibly pried out the button, and rasped the edges smooth" (pp. 437–438).

The late Sir Peter Buck (Te Rangi Hiroa), eminent New Zealand physician and anthropologist, delighted in boasting of the surgical knowledge of his Maori ancestors. Every adult male in this notoriously cannibalistic society had, he pointed out, a fuller and more detailed knowledge of human anatomy than that possessed by any modern European except specially trained physicians and surgeons. Moreover, it was Polynesian practitioners who first learned to expedite the healing of fractures in the long bones by inserting a stick pointed at both ends into the marrow on either side of the break, anticipating by centuries a recent "discovery" by a Danish scientist.

The pharmacopoeia of modern medicine, as is well known, includes numerous contributions from other cultures, notable among them being chaulmoogra oil (for the treatment of leprosy), coca and its derivative cocaine (as a pain suppressant), and quinine (as a specific for malaria). The great pharmaceutical companies are well aware of this fact. Some years ago, for example, the firm of Smith, Kline, and French offered a generous supplement to the research funds of members of the American Anthropological Association who would collect, preserve, and bring back from the field specimens of the plants reported by their informants to be used locally for medicinal purposes.

Most such early medical achievements are viewed, even by medical scientists, as discoveries of isolated cause-and-effect relationships, not as examples of broader categories of causation. We shall consequently find the ethnographic evidence of theories of natural causation rather unsatisfactory. Theories of supernatural causation, on the other hand, rest on a small number of basic postulates and hence lend themselves much more readily to classification.

I shall speak consistently of theories of illness rather than of disease, since the word "disease" has too narrow a connotation, suggesting primarily the communicable virus-borne or bacteria-borne ailments. "Illness" serves far better to connote the wider range of phenomena which we are interested in and which may be defined as embracing any impairment of health serious enough to arouse concern, whether it be due to communicable disease, psychosomatic disturbance, organic failure, aggressive assault, or alleged accident or supernatural interference.

Although death is a frequent result of illness, the causes of the two are not identical, and failure to distinguish them might lead to confusion. I, therefore, have decided to disregard whether or not the causes of illness might also eventuate in death and, consequently, have given less consideration to major calamities resulting in heavy fatalities, such as famine, floods, epidemics, earthquakes, and conflagrations, than to less spectacular ailments and injuries such as fevers, headache, nausea, wounds, fractures, and general malaise.

As a matter of fact, it is primarily to such lesser maladies and misadventures that primitive medicine became adapted. Populations were sparse, widely scattered, and relatively isolated. Infectious diseases could spread only with difficulty and tended to be localized in particular areas. "Under such circumstances," as stated elsewhere (Murdock 1952: 9), "a double evolutionary process takes place. Human beings gradually develop a relative immunity through a process of natural selection which eliminates the most susceptible strains in each generation. The disease microorganisms undergo an opposite evolutionary development which favors the less virulent strains; the more lethal strains kill their carriers and thus tend to be eliminated. In time, as a result of this dual process, the endemic diseases of a region become less dangerous to its inhabitants and the latter become less susceptible to the diseases."

In general, therefore, the ailments faced by early practitioners of the healing arts probably tended to be less serious, more responsive to simple remedies, and more likely to be functional or psychosomatic in character than might be expected. This would explain why medicine men in primitive societies have been less frequently herbalists or bonesetters, the forerunners of modern physicians and surgeons, than specialists in magical therapy, the ancestor of psychiatry.

Beginning about ten thousand years ago came a series of changes which completely altered the situation. Advances in agriculture and animal husbandry expanded the food supply. Technological inventions and increasing specialization and trade led to the expansion of population and its concentration in cities—conditions favorable to the spread of infection. Political conquest and state-building intensified this development, which reached its climax in the Discoveries Period, when explorers, colonists, traders, and missionaries combined to spread a host of communicable diseases from the limited areas where they were endemic to the rest of the world. Bubonic plague, cholera, smallpox, and typhus swept over the earth in successive epidemics and malaria, measles, syphilis, and tuberculosis took almost as heavy a toll.

Indigenous medicine men, of course, were helpless before this onslaught and suffered an irreparable deterioration in reputation. It would be ungenerous, however, to blame them for failure to cope with a situation which they were unprepared to meet and could not have predicted. Let us rather acknowledge the tremendous debt owed them for the solace, comfort, and material help they brought to suffering mankind over a period of perhaps two million years.

References Cited

Clements, F. E. Primitive Concepts of Disease. University of California Publications in American Archaeology and Ethnology 32: 185–252. 1932.

Murdock, G. P. Our Primitive Contemporaries. New York, 1934.

———. Anthropology and Its Contribution to Public Health. American Journal of Public Health 42: 7–11. 1952.

Tylor, E. B. Primitive Culture. 2 vols. London, 1871.

II

Theories of Natural Causation

The structure of the research, corrected by analysis of its findings, led to the ultimate establishment of a typology of theories of illness based on criteria derived in part from modern medical science and in part from anthropological experience. The first distinction to emerge was a basic dichotomy between theories of natural causation and theories of supernatural causation. Since medical science does not recognize the validity of supernatural causes, their classification depends exclusively on the anthropologist. For theories of natural causation, on the other hand, primary reliance must be placed on categories recognized by medical science, and the anthropologist's role is confined to ordering them in a framework suitable for comparative analysis with the least possible distortion of their scientific accuracy.

Our chief difficulty flows from the impossibility of knowing what the ultimate medical classification of illness causation may be and the consequent necessity of estimating its approximate parameters from the present state of scientific knowledge. I have thus allowed a modest leeway in assigning native theories to particular types of natural causation. For example, if a cause described in the ethnographic literature suggests emotional tension, I classify it under "stress," even though it fails to accord precisely with any recognized psychiatric definition. And if a society ascribes illness to invasion of the body by microorganisms, I classify the cause as "infection" even though the organisms as described do not particularly resemble germs. Such cases, moreover, may possibly reflect imperfect cultural borrowing from a more complex culture.

8

For purposes of classification I employ the following definition of theories of natural causation: *any theory, scientific or popular, which accounts for the impairment of health as a physiological consequence of some experience of the victim in a manner that would appear reasonable to modern medical science.* Five distinct types of theories which fall into this general category are distinguished and defined below.

Type 1: Infection. Defined as invasion of the victim's body by noxious microorganisms, with particular but not exclusive reference to the "germ theory of disease" deriving from the discoveries of Pasteur and Koch.

The only society in our world sample of 139 for which this is reported as the predominant theory of illness is the Japanese (#117), or more specifically the pinpointed inhabitants of southern Okayama prefecture. To be sure, there are doubtless a few others in the modern world which do not happen to be included in the sample. For only thirty-one other societies do the sources mention theories of this type as of even minor consequence, and in most of them the infecting organisms resemble worms or tiny insects rather than germs. The small number of societies reported to accept a theory of infection reflects both the recency of its scientific recognition and the very limited range of its diffusion. The Nama Hottentot (#1) and the Wodaabe Fulani (#25) hold ideas that are more sophisticated than most, since they actually practice certain rudimentary forms of immunization.

Type 2: Stress. Defined as exposure of the victim to either physical or psychic strain, such as overexertion, prolonged hunger or thirst, debilitating extremes of heat or cold, worry, fear, or the emotional disturbances which constitute the province of modern psychiatry.

Stress is reported as an important, though not dominant cause of illness in three societies—the Siamese (#76), Javanese (#83), and Ingalik (#122)—and as a lesser factor in approximately half the societies of the sample. The Marshallese (#108) and Tupinamba (#177), for example, ascribe illness to overexertion, especially during pregnancy; the Tiv (#16) and Rhade (#74), to overeating; the Javanese (#83) and Pawnee (#142) to anxiety; the inhabitants of

Uttar Pradesh (#63) and the Copper Eskimo (#124) to sharp changes in temperatures which trigger colds.

Type 3: Organic Deterioration. Defined as a decline in physical capacities attending the onset of old age, the earlier failure of particular organs such as the heart or kidneys, or the appearance of serious hereditary defects, often manifest at birth or in childhood.

Surprisingly, this seemingly obvious cause receives scant support from the ethnographic literature, being mentioned for only twenty-nine societies and never as an important determinant. The explanation doubtless resides in part in the widespread removal of defective infants by infanticide, in the very high mortality rates prevailing throughout most of the world, and in the slow and unspectacular nature of the aging process. In any event, it would seem as though most of mankind considers itself potentially immortal and is unable to conceive of the infirmities of old or middle age as being caused by anything other than the interference of some hostile agency or force.

Type 4: Accident. Defined as the suffering of some physical injury under circumstances which appear to exclude both intention on the part of the victim and suspicion of supernatural intervention.

Examples would include frostbite, burns, bites of snakes or insects, wounds from animal attacks, poisoning from unfamiliar mushrooms, cuts from the careless handling of weapons, and fractures from falls or vehicle collisions. Sometimes the triviality of the occurrence is decisive. The Mundurucu (#166), for example, attribute a cut to "mischance" if it is slight, but if it is serious they ascribe it to sorcery or evil spirits. The general tendency is to personalize the causation of what we term accidents and to attribute them to supernatural intervention. This presumably accounts for the rarity (only thirty-eight of the sample societies) with which the sources cite accident as a cause of illness—and never as a major one.

Type 5: Overt Human Aggression. Defined as the willful infliction of bodily injuries on another human being, as in violent quarrels, assault or mayhem, brawls, crimes of violence, warfare, and even attempted suicide (so-called "aggression turned inward").

Aggression is a universal human impulse, and its overt expression is likewise universal. No people can have failed to recognize it or have succeeded in disguising it by any amount of repression or rationalization. It is only through a sort of semantic misadventure—the widespread misuse of "disease" as a synonym for "illness"—that it has escaped recognition as a cause of illness and, indeed, as perhaps the most basic of all natural causes. Recognizing its obviousness from the outset, I gave the coders specific instructions, probably mistakenly as it now seems, not to record the evidence for it in the ethnographic sources. The aggressive acts occurring in fights, violent crime, and warfare indisputably impair the health of the victims, as any veterns' hospital can bear witness. And it is aggression of this type, not "disease," that man everywhere has generalized or projected to the supernatural beings he has created, with the result that the motive of aggression is central to many of the supernatural theories of illness to which attention will next be directed. Along with the phenomenon of death, it lies at the root of all supernatural ideology.

Table 1 presents the evidence on the incidence and relative importance of the natural causes of illness (other than the presumably universal one of overt human aggression) as reported for the 139 societies surveyed. The following numerical symbols are used: 3 for the predominant cause recognized by the society, 2 for an important auxiliary cause, 1 for a minor or relatively unimportant cause, 0 for the reported or strongly inferred absence of such a cause.

Table 1

Theories of the Natural Causation of Illness:
Incidence and Relative Importance

Society No.	Name	Theories of Infection	Theories of Stress	Theories of Deterioration	Theories of Accident
1.	Hottentot	1	0	1	1
2.	Bushmen	–	1	–	–
3.	Thonga	1	1	0	0
5.	Mbundu	0	1	0	0

Theories of Illness

Table 1 (continued)

No.	Society Name	Theories of Infection	Theories of Stress	Theories of Deterioration	Theories of Accident
6.	Suku	0	1	1	0
8.	Nyakyusa	1	1	0	0
9.	Hadza	1	0	0	0
11a.	Chagga	0	0	0	0
12.	Ganda	0	1	1	0
13.	Mbuti	0	1	1	1
14.	Mongo	0	0	0	1
15.	Banen	0	0	0	0
16.	Tiv	1	1	1	0
18.	Fon	0	1	0	0
19.	Ashanti	0	0	0	1
20.	Mende	–	–	1	–
21.	Wolof	0	0	0	1
23.	Tallensi	0	0	0	0
24.	Songhai	0	1	0	0
25.	Fulani	1	1	0	1
26.	Hausa	–	1	0	0
27.	Massa	0	0	0	0
28.	Azande	1	1	0	1
30.	Otoro	0	0	0	0
31.	Shilluk	0	0	0	1
32.	Mao	0	0	0	0
33.	Kaffa	0	0	0	0
34a.	Dorobo	1	0	0	0
36.	Somali	–	0	0	0
37.	Amhara	1	1	0	1
39.	Kenuzi	1	0	0	0
40.	Teda	–	1	0	0
41.	Tuareg	1	0	0	1
42.	Riffians	0	0	0	0
43.	Egyptians	0	1	0	0
44.	Hebrews	0	0	0	0
45.	Babylonians	0	1	0	0
46.	Rwala	–	0	0	0
47.	Turks	1	1	0	0

Table 1 (continued)

Society No.	Name	Theories of Infection	Theories of Stress	Theories of Deterioration	Theories of Accident
48.	Albanians	0	1	0	0
49.	Romans	–	1	0	1
50.	Basques	1	–	0	1
51a.	Scots	1	1	0	1
52.	Lapps	0	1	0	0
53.	Samoyed	1	1	0	0
57.	Kurd	0	0	0	0
60.	Gond	0	0	0	0
61.	Toda	0	–	–	–
63.	Uttar Pradesh	1	1	1	0
65.	Kazak	0	1	0	1
66.	Mongols	1	0	0	0
68.	Lepcha	1	1	1	0
69.	Garo	0	1	0	0
71.	Burmese	0	1	0	0
72.	Lamet	0	1	0	0
73.	Vietnamese	1	0	0	0
74.	Rhade	–	1	0	0
76.	Siamese	1	2	1	1
77.	Semang	0	1	0	0
78.	Nicobarese	0	0	0	0
79.	Andamanese	0	0	0	1
81.	Tanala	0	0	0	0
83.	Javanese	0	2	1	1
84.	Balinese	0	0	0	0
85.	Iban	0	0	0	0
86.	Badjau	0	1	1	0
87.	Toradja	1	1	1	1
89.	Alorese	0	1	0	0
90.	Tiwi	0	0	0	0
91.	Aranda	0	1	0	0
92.	Orokaiva	0	1	0	1
94.	Kapauku	0	0	0	0
95a.	Wogeo	0	1	0	0
96.	Manus	0	1	0	0

Theories of Illness

Table 1 (continued)

	Society	Theories of	Theories of	Theories of	Theories of
No.	Name	Infection	Stress	Deterioration	Accident
98.	Trobrianders	0	1	0	1
99.	Siuai	–	1	1	1
100.	Tikopia	0	1	1	0
102.	Fijians	0	0	1	1
103.	Ajie	0	0	0	0
105.	Marquesans	0	0	1	0
106.	Samoans	0	0	0	1
108.	Marshallese	1	1	1	1
109.	Trukese	0	1	0	0
111.	Palauans	0	0	1	0
112.	Ifugao	0	1	0	1
113.	Atayal	0	0	0	0
115.	Manchu	0	0	0	1
117.	Japanese	3	1	1	0
118.	Ainu	1	1	1	1
120.	Yukaghir	0	1	0	0
121.	Chukchee	0	1	0	1
122.	Ingalik	1	2	1	1
123.	Aleut	1	–	0	0
124.	Copper Eskimo	0	1	0	0
126.	Micmac	0	1	0	0
127.	Saulteaux	0	0	0	1
128.	Slave	0	0	0	0
129.	Kaska	0	0	0	0
131.	Haida	0	0	0	0
132.	Bellacoola	0	1	1	0
133.	Twana	0	1	0	1
134.	Yurok	0	1	0	0
135.	Pomo	0	0	–	0
137.	Wadadika	0	1	1	0
138.	Klamath	1	0	0	0
139.	Kutenai	–	1	–	–
141a.	Crow	0	0	0	0
142.	Pawnee	–	0	1	0
143.	Omaha	0	0	0	0

Table 1 (continued)

Society No.	Name	Theories of Infection	Theories of Stress	Theories of Deterioration	Theories of Accident
144.	Huron	0	–	0	0
147.	Comanche	0	1	0	0
148.	Chiricahua	0	1	1	1
149.	Zuni	0	0	1	0
150.	Havasupai	0	1	0	0
153.	Aztec	0	0	0	0
154.	Popoluca	1	1	–	–
155.	Quiche	0	1	0	0
156.	Miskito	0	1	0	0
158.	Cuna	0	1	0	1
159.	Goajiro	0	1	0	0
160.	Haitians	0	0	0	0
162.	Warrau	0	0	0	0
165.	Saramacca	0	1	0	0
166.	Mundurucu	0	0	0	1
167.	Cubeo	0	0	0	0
169.	Jivaro	1	1	1	1
170.	Amahuaca	0	1	0	0
171.	Inca	0	0	0	0
172.	Aymara	0	1	1	1
173.	Siriono	1	1	0	1
175a.	Bororo	0	0	0	0
176.	Timbira	0	0	0	0
177.	Tupinamba	0	1	0	0
179a.	Caraja	0	1	0	0
180.	Aweikoma	0	0	0	0
182.	Lengua	1	1	0	0
184.	Mapuche	0	–	0	0
185.	Tehuelche	0	0	1	0
186.	Yahgan	1	0	0	1

With the striking exception of overt human aggression and the partial exception of stress, the natural causes of illness have received remarkably little attention in the ethnographic literature. While this may possibly reflect a stronger interest in the supernatural among anthropologists, I strongly suspect that the real strength of interest resides more among the peoples studied than among those who study them.

At this point mention should be made of a category of theories of illness which occupy a sort of twilight zone between those of natural and supernatural causation. They occur mainly in situations where confident acceptance of a particular therapeutic technique has generated a consistent but often incompletely formulated theory of causation. Familiar contemporary examples include such practices as acupuncture, chiropractic, osteopathy, and various versions of faith healing. None is generally accepted by medical scientists, and none has substantial experimental support, yet there are seemingly valid grounds for assuming that they are not wholly lacking in therapeutic effectiveness. A common characteristic is the organization of their supporters in cultlike groups, often with charismatic leadership as in India. They are no less frequent in simple than in complex societies, as witness the widespread prevalence of "medicine societies" among North American Indians. No attempt is made herewith to deal with theories of this sort because (1) they are derivative rather than primary and hence usually imprecisely defined; (2) scientific grounds are insufficient to classify them as theories of natural causation; and (3) their connotations are not necessarily supernatural though they often have religious overtones.

III

Theories of Supernatural Causation

Analysis of the findings of the study, in conjunction with leads from the literature of anthropology, led to the isolation of eight additional types of theories concerned with the causation of illness. These have little in common other than that they all rest on supernatural assumptions which modern medical science does not recognize as valid. They do, however, fall into three readily distinguishable groups, each of which is capable of separate definition: (1) theories of mystical causation, (2) theories of animistic causation, and (3) theories of magical causation.

Theories of Mystical Causation

These may be defined as *any theory which accounts for the impairment of health as the automatic consequence of some act or experience of the victim mediated by some putative impersonal causal relationship rather than by the intervention of a human or supernatural being.* These theories may perhaps be characterized most readily as those which accord more closely with the animatism or preanimism of R. R. Marett (1909) than with the animism of E. B. Tylor (1871). Four specific types of causation fall into this category.

Type 6: Fate. Defined as the ascription of illness to astrological influences, individual predestination, or personified ill luck.

Fate is reported to be a major determinant of illness only among the ancient Romans (#49). Its twenty-eight other occurrences also tend to be concentrated in societies of considerable complexity, for

17

example, the Ganda (#12), Fon (#18), Ashanti (#19), Egyptians (#43), Turks (#47), Uttar Pradesh (#63), Burmese (#71), Vietnamese (#73), Siamese (#76), Javanese (#83), and Aztec (#153).

Type 7: Ominous Sensations. Defined as the experiencing of particularly potent kinds of dreams, sights, sounds, or other sensations which are believed to cause and not merely to portend illness.

Examples in our sample include dreaming of a recently deceased relative among the Massa (#27), looking at one's own shadow among the Egyptians (#43), and imagining the metamorphosis of a deer into a woman among the Pawnee (#142). Such causes, rarely of more than very minor importance, are reported for thirty-seven of the societies surveyed.

Type 8: Contagion. Defined as coming into contact with some purportedly polluting object, substance, or person.

This mystical cause, which roughly parallels the natural cause of infection, is attested for forty-nine societies. In one, the Thonga (#3), it is reported to be a major though not the predominant cause of illness. Among a variety of sources of contagion by far the most widespread are (1) menstrual blood or a menstruating woman and (2) the corpse of a deceased person or some object associated therewith. The former preponderates in North America; the latter, in Africa. Leprosy provides an interesting special case. Though it is recognized by modern medicine as a mildly infectious disease, the avoidance of its victims has closer parallels with that of such purportedly polluting categories of people as the "untouchables" of India.

Type 9: Mystical Retribution. Defined as acts in violation of some taboo or moral injunction when conceived as causing illness directly rather than through the mediation of some offended or punitive supernatural being.

In the literature this has sometimes been called the taboo violation theory. It is reported as the predominant theory of illness among the Thonga (#3), Hadza (#9), Nkundo Mongo (#14), Otoro (#30), and Kaska (#129); as of substantial but secondary importance in thirty-four other societies; as present but unimportant in seventy-one;

and as apparently absent in only twenty-nine. The major categories of relevant taboos are listed below in the order of frequency with which they are reported in this connection:

Food taboos, including drinking prohibitions
Sex taboos, for example, against incest or adultery
Etiquette taboos, that is, breaches of appropriate behavior toward kinsmen, strangers, or social superiors
Ritual taboos, that is, breaches of appropriate behavior toward the supernatural
Property taboos, for example, against trespass or theft
Verbal taboos, for example, against blasphemy or the use of forbidden words

Theories of Animistic Causation

These may be defined as *any theory which ascribes the impairment of health to the behavior of some personalized supernatural entity— a soul, ghost, spirit, or god.* They accord particularly closely with the doctrine of animism set forth by E. B. Tylor. Two distinct types of illness causation fall into this category.

Type 10: Soul Loss. Defined as the ascription of illness to the voluntary and more-than-temporary departure of the victim's soul from his body.

This is to be distinguished from the involuntary departure or capture of the soul through an act of sorcery. Most simpler religions postulate that every human being has an insubstantial double or soul which normally resides within his body but is capable of leaving temporarily to have the experiences perceived in dreams and which departs permanently at death to lead a differentiated afterlife. If death is the consequence of the soul's final departure, it is logical to conclude that a somewhat less prolonged absence may cause its owner to fall ill.

Soul loss is reported as a minor cause of illness in thirty-seven of the sample societies. It ranks second in importance, however, in a society that I studied at first hand (Murdock 1965), the Tenino Indians of Oregon. The Tenino normally ascribe illness to sorcery by spirit possession, and the shaman ascertains the identity of the intruder by sending a special diagnostic guardian spirit into the patient's body on an exploratory mission. Occasionally what it finds is not the presence of a malignant intrusive spirit which must be exorcised but the absence of the patient's own soul. This is particularly likely to occur when the patient has recently lost a dear one by death—a beloved spouse or child—and has become so depressed and despondent that his soul abandons its body to follow the departed soul of the deceased to the spirit world. To meet such an emergency, every Tenino shaman has one human ghost among his retinue of guardian spirits. This he dispatches to the spirit world with orders to return with the patient's wandering soul, which if received in time he restores to the patient's body, thereby assuring recovery.

Type 11: Spirit Aggression. Defined as the attribution of illness to the direct hostile, arbitrary, or punitive action of some malevolent or affronted supernatural being.

This is distinguished from overt human aggression (Type 5 above) because the suspected aggressor is a ghost, spirit, or deity rather than a human being and from instances of magical causation (Type 12 below) where the supernatural being merely acts on the instigation, or as the agent, of a human aggressor. Spirit aggression is the most common and widespread of all the types of supernatural causation, as might be expected from the fact that it represents the most direct and obvious projection from overt human aggression. It is reported as the predominant cause of illness in seventy-eight of the sample societies, as an important secondary cause in forty, and as a rare or minor cause in nineteen. It is unreported or absent in only two societies—the Hadza (#9) and Slave (#128). The principal types of supernatural aggressors are identified as nature spirits, disease demons, or other lesser divinities in 104 instances; departed ancestors or kinsmen in 33; ghosts in 32; and higher deities or gods in 22.

Theories of Magical Causation

These may be defined as *any theory which ascribes illness to the covert action of an envious, affronted, or malicious human being who employs magical means to injure his victims.* Two distinct types of illness causation fall into this category.

Type 12: Sorcery. Defined as the ascription of the impairment of health to the aggressive use of magical techniques by a human being, either independently or with the assistance of a specialized magician or shaman.

Sorcery is reported to be the principal cause of illness in twenty-eight of the sample societies, an important subsidiary cause in forty-four, and a rare or minor cause in fifty, with negative or insufficient evidence in seventeen. In order of their worldwide frequency, the magical techniques found to be most widely used are the following:

Verbal spells, prayers, or curses

Object intrusion, that is, ostensible projection of foreign objects into the victim's body

Divers techniques of contagious magic

Rites of exuvial magic performed over hair, nail parings, excreta, or discarded clothing of the victim

Administration of presumptive poisons, commonly with only imaginary effectiveness

Divers techniques of imitative magic

Dispatch of alien spirits to possess the victim's body

Theft or capture of the victim's soul

Type 13: Witchcraft. Defined as the ascription of the impairment of health to the suspected voluntary or involuntary aggressive action of a member of a special class of human beings believed to be endowed with a special power and propensity for evil.

Witches are especially prone to envy. They employ various techniques, but by far the most common is that called *iettatura* in Italian and evil eye in English. Witchcraft is reported as the predominant cause of illness in nine societies, as an important secondary cause in eighteen, and as a minor cause in twenty-seven. It is practically universal in the Circum-Mediterranean region but surprisingly rare elsewhere in the world. The distinction between witchcraft and sorcery,

Theories of Illness

difficult to comprehend for individuals lacking actual experience with either practice, will be made clear in Chapter VIII.

The incidence and relative importance of the various theories of the supernatural causation of illness, as reported for the sample societies, are presented in Table 2. The symbols are the same as in Table 1: 3 for the predominant cause recognized by the society, 2 for an important auxiliary cause, 1 for a minor or relatively unimportant cause, 0 for the reported or strongly inferred absence of such a cause.

Table 2

Theories of the Supernatural Causation of Illness:
Incidence and Relative Importance

No.	Society Name	Fate	Ominous Sens.	Contagion	Mystical Retribution	Soul Loss	Spirit Aggression	Sorcery	Witchcraft
1.	Hottentot	0	0	0	1	0	3	2	0
2.	Bushmen	0	0	1	1	0	3	0	0
3.	Thonga	1	0	2	3	0	2	1	2
5.	Mbundu	0	0	0	1	0	2	2	0
6.	Suku	0	0	0	2	0	1	2	2
8.	Nyakyusa	0	0	1	1	0	2	2	3
9.	Hadza	0	0	1	3	0	0	1	0
11a.	Chagga	0	0	0	1	0	2	3	1
12.	Ganda	1	0	1	2	0	2	2	0
13.	Mbuti	0	0	0	1	0	3	1	0
14.	Mongo	0	0	0	3	0	1	1	0
15.	Banen	0	1	0	2	0	1	2	2
16	Tiv	0	0	0	2	0	1	0	3
18.	Fon	1	0	1	1	0	2	2	0
19.	Ashanti	1	1	0	1	1	3	1	2
20.	Mende	0	1	1	2	0	2	2	1
21.	Wolof	0	0	0	2	0	2	1	3
23.	Tallensi	0	0	0	2	0	3	1	0
24.	Songhai	1	1	0	1	0	2	1	2
25.	Fulani	1	0	1	1	0	2	2	0
26.	Hausa	0	1	0	1	0	3	1	1

Table 2 (continued)

Society No.	Name	Fate	Ominous Sens.	Contagion	Mystical Retribution	Soul Loss	Spirit Aggression	Sorcery	Witchcraft
27.	Massa	0	–	0	0	0	3	2	0
28.	Azande	0	1	1	1	0	1	2	3
30.	Otoro	0	0	0	3	0	1	2	0
31.	Shilluk	0	0	0	1	0	3	1	2
32.	Mao	0	0	0	0	0	2	0	2
33.	Kaffa	0	0	0	0	0	3	0	2
34a.	Dorobo	0	0	0	0	0	3	0	1
36.	Somali	0	0	0	0	0	3	1	1
37.	Amhara	0	0	0	1	0	3	1	2
39.	Kenuzi	0	0	0	0	0	2	1	3
40.	Teda	0	0	0	1	0	2	1	3
41.	Tuareg	0	0	0	1	0	3	0	1
42.	Riffians	0	1	0	0	0	1	2	2
43.	Egyptians	–	1	0	2	0	2	0	2
44.	Hebrews	0	0	0	0	0	2	0	3
45.	Babylonians	0	0	0	2	0	3	2	1
46.	Rwala	1	1	0	0	–	2	1	2
47.	Turks	1	0	0	0	0	3	0	1
48.	Albanians	0	0	0	0	0	2	2	3
49.	Romans	2	0	0	0	0	2	2	1
50.	Basques	0	–	0	1	0	3	1	2
51a.	Scots	0	0	0	0	0	2	1	2
52.	Lapps	0	1	1	1	0	3	2	0
53.	Samoyed	0	0	1	1	0	3	0	0
57.	Kurd	0	0	0	0	0	2	1	3
60.	Gond	0	1	0	1	0	2	3	0
61.	Toda	0	0	1	1	0	3	2	2
63.	Uttar Pradesh	1	0	1	1	0	3	1	1
65.	Kazak	0	0	0	0	0	3	1	1
66.	Mongols	0	0	0	0	0	3	1	0
68.	Lepcha	1	1	1	1	1	3	1	1
69.	Garo	1	0	0	1	1	3	1	0
71.	Burmese	1	0	0	1	1	3	2	0

Table 2 (continued)

No.	Society Name	Fate	Ominous Sens.	Contagion	Mystical Retribution	Soul Loss	Spirit Aggression	Sorcery	Witchcraft
72.	Lamet	0	0	0	0	0	2	1	0
73.	Vietnamese	1	0	0	2	1	3	2	0
74.	Rhade	0	1	0	0	0	3	1	0
76.	Siamese	1	0	0	2	1	3	1	1
77.	Semang	0	1	0	2	0	3	1	0
78.	Nicobarese	0	0	0	1	1	3	0	1
79.	Andamanese	0	1	1	1	1	3	1	0
81.	Tanala	0	1	0	1	1	3	2	0
83.	Javanese	1	0	0	1	0	3	1	0
84.	Balinese	1	0	1	0	0	3	2	0
85.	Iban	1	0	1	2	1	3	1	0
86.	Badjau	1	0	0	2	0	3	1	0
87.	Toradja	1	1	1	2	1	3	2	1
89.	Alorese	0	0	0	2	1	3	1	0
90.	Tiwi	0	0	0	2	0	3	1	0
91.	Aranda	0	0	0	2	0	2	3	1
92.	Orokaiva	0	0	–	1	0	3	2	0
94.	Kapauku	0	0	1	2	0	3	1	0
95a.	Wogeo	0	0	1	2	0	1	3	0
96.	Manus	0	0	0	0	0	3	1	0
98.	Trobrianders	0	0	1	1	0	1	3	2
99.	Siuai	1	0	0	1	1	2	3	0
100.	Tikopia	0	0	0	1	0	3	2	0
102.	Fijians	1	0	1	1	0	2	3	0
103.	Ajie	0	0	0	1	–	3	1	0
105.	Marquesans	0	0	1	0	1	3	2	0
106.	Samoans	0	0	1	1	–	3	2	0
108.	Marshallese	0	1	1	2	1	3	2	0
109.	Trukese	0	0	1	1	1	3	2	0
111.	Palauans	–	0	1	1	0	3	1	0
112.	Ifugao	0	0	0	1	0	3	1	1
113.	Atayal	1	0	0	1	0	3	0	0
115.	Manchu	0	0	1	1	0	3	0	0

Table 2 (continued)

No.	Society Name	Fate	Ominous Sens.	Contagion	Mystical Retribution	Soul Loss	Spirit Aggression	Sorcery	Witchcraft
117.	Japanese	–	0	0	0	0	2	0	0
118.	Ainu	0	1	1	1	1	3	2	0
120.	Yukaghir	0	0	0	1	1	3	1	0
121.	Chukchee	0	1	1	2	0	3	2	0
122.	Ingalik	0	1	1	2	1	3	1	0
123.	Aleut	0	0	1	1	0	3	1	0
124.	Copper Eskimo	0	0	0	0	1	3	1	0
126.	Micmac	0	0	1	1	1	3	1	2
127.	Saulteaux	0	0	0	2	0	1	3	0
128.	Slave	0	0	1	1	0	0	3	0
129.	Kaska	0	0	0	3	0	1	2	0
131.	Haida	0	0	0	1	1	1	3	1
132.	Bellacoola	1	0	0	2	1	3	2	0
133.	Twana	0	0	1	1	1	1	3	0
134.	Yurok	1	1	1	1	1	1	3	0
135.	Pomo	0	1	1	2	1	2	2	0
137.	Wadadika	0	0	1	1	0	3	2	0
138.	Klamath	0	1	0	2	0	1	3	0
139.	Kutenai	0	1	0	2	0	2	2	0
141a.	Crow	0	0	0	2	0	3	2	0
142.	Pawnee	0	1	0	1	0	1	3	0
143.	Omaha	0	0	1	2	0	1	2	0
144.	Huron	0	0	0	1	0	3	2	0
147.	Comanche	0	0	0	1	0	3	1	2
148.	Chiricahua	0	1	1	1	0	2	3	0
149.	Zuni	0	0	0	2	–	2	3	1
150.	Havasupai	1	1	1	2	1	3	1	1
153.	Aztec	1	1	0	1	0	2	3	1
154.	Popoluca	0	1	0	2	0	2	3	1
155.	Quiche	1	0	0	0	0	3	2	0
156.	Miskito	0	1	0	1	0	3	2	0
158.	Cuna	1	1	–	2	0	3	1	1
159.	Goajiro	0	0	0	1	0	3	1	1

Table 2 (continued)

Society No.	Name	Fate	Ominous Sens.	Contagion	Mystical Retribution	Soul Loss	Spirit Aggression	Sorcery	Witchcraft
160.	Haitians	0	0	0	1	0	3	2	1
162.	Warrau	0	0	1	1	1	2	3	0
165.	Saramacca	0	0	0	1	1	3	2	0
166.	Mundurucu	0	0	1	0	0	2	3	1
167.	Cubeo	0	0	0	1	0	1	3	0
169.	Jivaro	0	0	0	1	0	2	3	1
170.	Amahuaca	0	1	0	1	0	2	3	0
171.	Inca	0	0	1	0	1	3	2	0
172.	Aymara	0	1	1	1	1	3	2	0
173.	Siriono	0	0	1	1	1	3	0	0
175a.	Bororo	0	0	1	2	0	3	0	0
176.	Timbira	0	1	–	1	0	1	3	0
177.	Tupinamba	0	–	0	0	0	3	1	0
179a.	Caraja	0	0	0	0	0	2	3	0
180.	Aweikoma	0	0	1	1	0	3	0	0
182.	Lengua	–	1	0	1	2	2	3	0
184.	Mapuche	0	0	0	1	0	2	3	0
185.	Tehuelche	0	–	1	0	0	3	1	0
186.	Yahgan	0	1	0	1	0	2	3	0

A comparison of Tables 1 and 2 strongly reinforces the conclusion that supernatural causes of illness far outweigh natural causes in the belief systems of the world's peoples. Especially prominent and widespread are, in rank order, the animistic theory of spirit aggression, the magical theory of sorcery, and the mystical theory of retribution for taboo violations. Also significant, though with a more restricted distribution, are beliefs ascribing illness to the baleful influence of witches.

The early chapters of this book have defined, exemplified, and classified the types of theories of illness encountered in surveying a representative sample of the world's best-described societies. Remaining to be considered are the distribution of these concepts over the earth's surface and the scientific reasons, insofar as these can be ascertained, for the emergence and prominence of the most widespread theories of supernatural causation. Certain important problems of theory and method, however, must receive prior attention.

References Cited

Marett, R. R. The Threshold of Religion. London, 1909.
Murdock, G. P. Tenino Shamanism. Ethnology 4: 165–171. 1965.
Tylor, E. B. Primitive Culture. 2 vols. London, 1871.

IV

Behavioral Science and
the Comparative Ethnographic Method

In analyzing theories of illness, this study employs the time-honored method of cross-cultural comparison. Its theoretical orientation, however, is that of contemporary behavioral science, which in recent years has achieved a notable rapprochement between anthropology, psychology, and sociology. As theory alters over time, method must necessarily keep pace. A brief review of the history of the comparative ethnographic method will clarify the changes that have taken place.

Around the middle of the eighteenth century a group of Scottish scholars, notably Adam Ferguson, David Hume, Lord Kames (Henry Home), John Millar, and Adam Smith, growing discontented with the limitations of philosophy and history, began to explore areas of human behavior that had previously been ignored. Influenced by the changes wrought by the Industrial Revolution at home and by the expanded world horizons resulting from the Discoveries Period, they showed an interest in aspects of behavior other than warfare and state-building—particularly economics, technology, language, family organization, and religion—and sought in such practices among other peoples clues to the origin of their own institutions. Thus came into being, in a momentous twin birth, both the scientific approach to human behavior and the comparative ethnographic method.

This innovative movement gained enormous impetus with the appearance of Darwin's *On the Origin of the Species* in 1859. In the following half century (1860–1910) there emerged and became differentiated, out of the matrix of scholars using the comparative method,

28

all the disciplines now recognized as behavioral sciences. The movement became one of the dominant intellectual conncerns of the entire civilized world, as can be indicated by a selected list of works by its principal scholars:

Atkinson, J. J. Primal Law. London, 1908.

Bachofen, J. J. Das Mutterrecht. Stuttgart, 1861.

Bartels, M. Die Medicin der Naturvölker. Leipzig, 1893.

Bastian, A. Der Mensch in der Geschichte. 3 vols. Leipzig, 1860.

Crawley, A. E. The Mystic Rose. London, 1902.

Dargun, L. Mutterrecht und Vaterrecht. Leipzig, 1892.

Engels, F. Der Ursprung der Familie, des Privateigentums und des Staates. Zurich, 1884.

Frazer, J. G. The Golden Bough. 2 vols. London, 1890.

Giraud-Teulon, A. Les origines du mariage et de la famille. Geneva, 1884.

Gomme, G. L. Ethnology in Folklore. London, 1892.

Grosse, E. Die Formen der Familie and die Formen der Wirthschaft. Freiburg, 1896.

Hahn, E. Die Haustiere und ihre Beziehungen zur Wirtschaft des Menschen. Leipzig, 1896.

Hellwald, F. von. Kulturgeschichte in ihrer natürlichen Entwickelung. 2 vols. Augsburg, 1896.

Howard, G. E. A History of Matrimonial Institutions. 3 vols. Chicago, 1904.

Kohler, J. Zur Urgeschichte der Ehe. Stuttgart, 1897.

Kropotkin, P. Mutual Aid. London, 1902.

Lang, A. Myth, Ritual and Religion. 2 vols. London, 1887.

Legouvé, E. Histoire morale des femmes. Paris, 1874.

Lehmann, A. Aberglaube und Zauberei. Stuttgart, 1898.

Letourneau, C. La sociologie d'après l'ethnographie. Paris, 1880.

Levy-Bruhl, L. Les fonctions mentales dans les sociétés inférieures. Paris, 1910.

Lippert, J. Kulturgeschichte der Menschheit in ihrem organischen Aufbau. 2 vols. Stuttgart, 1886.

Lubbock, J. (Lord Avebury). The Origin of Civilisation and the Primitive Condition of Man. London, 1870.

McLennan, J. F. Studies in Ancient History. London, 1876.

Maine, H. S. Ancient Law. London, 1861.

Marett, R. R. The Threshold of Religion. London, 1900.

Mason, O. T. The Origins of Invention. London, 1895.

Morgan, L. H. Ancient Society. New York, 1877.

Müller, J. Das sexuelle Leben der Naturvölker. Leipzig, 1906.

Nieboer, H. J. Slavery as an Industrial System. The Hague, 1900.

Ploss, H. H. Das Kind in Brauch und Sitte der Völker. Leipzig, 1906.

Post, A. H. Grundriss der ethnologischer Jurisprudenz. 2 vols. Oldenburg, 1894–95.

Schurtz, H. Alterklassen und Männerbünde. Berlin, 1902.

Spencer, H. The Principles of Sociology. 3 vols. New York, 1876–96.

Starcke, C. N. The Primitive Family. New York, 1889.

Steinmetz, S. R. Ethnologische Studien zur ersten Entwicklung der Strafe. 2 vols. Leiden, 1894.

Sumner, W. G. Folkways. Boston, 1906.

Thomas, W. I. Sex and Society. Chicago, 1907.

Tylor, E. B. Primitive Culture. 2 vols. London, 1871.

Van Gennep, L. Les rites de passage. Paris, 1909.

Vierkandt, A. Naturvölker und Kulturvölker. Leipzig, 1896.

Webster, H. Primitive Secret Societies. New York, 1908.

Westermarck, E. A. The History of Human Marriage. London, 1889.

Wilutzky, P. Vorgeschichte des Rechts. 3 vols. Breslau, 1903.

Wundt, W. Völkerpsychologie. 10 vols. Leipzig, 1900–20.

The above works and their ilk constituted the bulk of the intellectual fare of behavioral scientists when I was taking my first courses in anthropology, psychology, and sociology as an undergraduate in 1917 and 1918. I still find their authors impressive in their extraordinary international and interdisciplinary unity. They all adhered to the comparative ethnographic method. Nearly all were thoroughly familiar with the publications of the others. With the exception of an occasional critic, they tended to reach conclusions essentially consistent with one another. Under the influence of the unquestioned scientific leadership of Germany during this period, they exhibited an average level of scholarship appreciably higher that that achieved by their successors ever since. But they were mainly "armchair scholars" since even the anthropologists among them had scarcely begun as yet to engage in first-hand field research. The sources they used were largely reports by early explorers, travelers, missionaries, and colonial administrators, and do not even remotely compare in quality or completeness to most of those we cite in the Appendix.

I have observed closely the subsequent developments in the behavioral sciences. What happened part way into the twentieth century was a rapid and almost unanimous repudiation of the comparative ethnographic method. A relentless attack on the early comparativists was launched by Franz Boas (1896), who called attention to serious errors in their methodology. One such mistake occurred in generalizing Darwin's contribution from the biological to the cultural level, in which the concept of evolution was distorted from a divergent or branching process analogous to a tree to a unilineal stepwise process analogous to a ladder. Specifically, the evolutionists postulated a series of stages of development, from savagery through barbarism to civilization, through which all peoples were assumed to have passed. The mistake should have been obvious from the manifest differences in the apparent course of cultural development in Africa, Eurasia, and the New World, but it lingered on, supported by European ethnocentric prejudice, until it was finally quashed by Julian Steward (1955).

A second and even more serious error resulted from the way the comparative materials were used. The procedure usually followed was to examine many ethnographic sources for passages that seemed pertinent to the subject under investigation, to excerpt these and file them according to a predetermined system of classification along with similar cullings from other cultures, and ultimately to scrutinize the packets of such extracts topic by topic in order to make generalizations from them. All too frequently the conclusions, far from being actual inductions from the data, merely reflected assumptions implicit in the system of classification.

The Boasian strictures encountered remarkably little resistance. Within a few years they were almost universally accepted, and both evolutionist theory and the comparative method became virtually extinct in the behavioral sciences. But the baby had been thrown out with the bath water. Almost immediately the behavioral sciences lost their unity and underwent fragmentation. The separate disciplines lost contact with and respect for one another and individually disintegrated into warring "schools." I vividly recall, for example, the utter contempt openly manifested by my principal graduate mentor for Boasian anthropology, Freudian and behaviorist psychology, and the dominant schools in American, French, and German sociology. Provincialism and mutual distrust reigned supreme.

One compensating trend, however, was shortly to appear in anthropology. Under the stimulus of Boas and Bronislaw Malinowski fieldwork came to be expected of all young anthropologists. They spent longer and longer periods in the field and increasingly acquired the competence to converse freely with informants in their native language. And they adopted signficant refinements in field techniques, ranging from the admirable genealogical method to modern ethnoscience. Today ethnographic work of the highest quality is not confined to one or a few nations or schools of thought but is being produced in many countries by talented amateurs as well as skilled professionals.

Ironically, as ethnography improved there were proportionately fewer scholars willing to read it. Psychologists and sociologists were no longer interested. Anthropologists tended increasingly to confine their browsing to the few tribes studied by themselves and their more congenial colleagues. Students at all levels avoided ethnographic courses and readings, and became obsessed with the illusory notion that professional advancement is more readily achievable by virtuosity in theory than by command of data.

In the meantime, fragmentation in the behavioral sciences proceeded apace. So-called "historical" schools emerged under Boas and Alfred Kroeber in the United States and in other guises in England and central Europe. They all abandoned both science and the comparative method. Separate schools of "social anthropology" developed in France and Great Britain. These rejected both psychology and the comparative method and deluded themselves in postulating a new and mythical kind of "social facts" (see Murdock 1971). To be sure, they produced ethnographies of high quality, but so did historical anthropologists of several persuasions, for example, Martin Gusinde and Leslie Spier. The disciples of A. R. Radcliffe-Brown in England, more provincial than those of Claude Lévi-Strauss across the Channel, contemptuously refrained from examining either the descriptive or the theoretical writings of those whom Malinowski acidly dubbed "the Boasinine school."

In the 1930s the tide of negativism began to turn. A number of leading American anthropologists, headed by Ralph Linton, A. I. Hallowell, Clyde Kluckhohn, Margaret Mead, and John Gillin, paid heed for the first time to their colleagues in psychology and sociology, modified their own views accordingly, and laid the foundations for a more eclectic orientation in their discipline. In the Institute of Human Relations at Yale University scholars in several fields sponsored a creative synthesis in which behavioral psychology provided the basic theory, cultural anthropology its magnificent body of ethnographic data, and sociology certain aspects of perspective and methodology. This movement was continued at Harvard University with the establishment of the Department of Social Relations.

At this time Roland B. Dixon of Harvard and Richard Thurnwald of the University of Berlin stood almost alone among anthropologists of note in insisting on the high value of a knowledge of world ethnography. In 1937 I joined them by founding at the Institute of Human Relations the forerunner of the present Human Relations Area Files, a powerful instrument for making readily accessible to scholars an organized body of ethnographic data on a sample of the world's most fully described cultures. Today sets of these files are available in more than two hundred institutions of learning in the United States and abroad, and their use is rapidly expanding. Psychologists and sociologists, as well as anthropologists, are now returning in increasing numbers to the utilization of ethnographic data. Behavioral science and the comparative method, once joined prematurely for half a century and then violently parted for decades, have been brought together in what appears to be a much more harmonious and productive synthesis.

I shall now specify the procedures adopted in this volume to meet the legitimate criticisms of the earlier comparative method and to conform with the newer interdisciplinary standards of modern cross-cultural research.

Definitions

The first step in a comparative study is to define precisely those aspects of the subject under investigation whose relationships one intends to examine. I have already defined in Chapters II and III the types of theories of illness whose geographical distributions and cultural concomitants will be explored. Such definitions must, of course, be carefully pretested against a sample of the case materials to ascertain their adequacy and correct their initial deficiencies.

Sampling

Early users of the comparative ethnographic method drew their materials from as wide a range of descriptive sources as their scholarly interests dictated and their language competence permitted. It has proved increasingly impossible, however, to exhaust the descriptive literature, which keeps expanding at an accelerating rate. Sketchy regional surveys have consequently given way to fuller accounts of individual cultures, with stress being increasingly laid on studying societies of maximal geographic and cultural diversity. Ultimately most comparativists have reached tacit agreement that their samples should be drawn from, and be reasonably representative of, a "universe" consisting of all human societies for whose cultures relatively full descriptions are available.

One acceptable procedure is to select a sample from this universe by some random method. The most widely used such "probability sample" is the so-called "blue ribbon sample" of the Human Relations Area Files (HRAF) (see R. O. Lagacé 1977). Although invaluable to novices in cross-cultural research and unquestionably capable of yielding valid results in the simple testing of scientific hypotheses, probability samples reveal certain inherent defects. For example, since the composition of a probability sample is dependent upon chance, it necessarily produces a spotty and irregular geographical coverage and thus militates against the discovery of areal and regional distributions of the kind sought in Chapter V.

Preference is consequently given herewith to the use of a stratified sample, a more accurate and sophisticated type of sample modeled on those employed in the leading public-opinion polls. This sample was developed after prolonged research with assistance from Douglas R. White (see Murdock and White 1969). It involved the analysis of nearly 1,300 disparate cultures, their grouping into 186 sampling provinces, and the selection of a representative society from each.

Since a sample employed for a single study has only limited usefulness, my former associates at the University of Pittsburgh and I have produced eight comparative studies[1] employing the same standard sample of 186 societies, with only an occasional deletion or substitution:

Barry, H., III, L. Josephson, E. Lauer, and C. Marshall. Traits Inculcated in Childhood. Ethnology 15: 83–114. 1976.

Barry, H., III, and L. M. Paxson. Infancy and Early Childhood. Ethnology 10: 466–508. 1971.

Murdock, G. P., and D. O. Morrow. Subsistence Economy and Supportive Practices. Ethnology 9: 302–330. 1970.

Murdock, G. P., and C. Provost. Factors in the Division of Labor by Sex. Ethnology 12: 203–225. 1973.

Murdock, G. P., and C. Provost. Measurement of Cultural Complexity. Ethnology 12: 379–392. 1973.

Murdock, G. P., and S. F. Wilson. Settlement Patterns and Community Organization. Ethnology 11: 254–295. 1972.

Roberts, J. M. Belief in the Evil Eye in World Perspective. The Evil Eye, ed. C. Moloney, pp. 223–278. New York, 1976.

Tuden, A., and C. Marshall. Political Organization. Ethnology 11: 436–466. 1972.

The variables in any one of these studies can readily be intercorrelated with those in the others—including the ones in this volume—making possible a wide variety of statistical tests.

Owing to pressure of time, curtailment of funds, and frequent insufficiency of information on illness, the size of the sample for the present study has been reduced about 25 percent to 139. Though impaired by the elimination of certain important cultures, notably the contemporary Russians (#54) and the Chekiang Chinese (#114), the reduced sample shows a reasonably uniform geographical distribution over the earth.

One serious deficiency of the HRAF probability sample is its exclusion of all the societies of antiquity known to us through historical scholarship, such as the Hebrews (#44), Babylonians (#45), and Romans (#49) in our own sample and even of such societies as the Aztec (#153) and Inca (#171), to the knowledge of which historians have made a major contribution. A second is its failure to include even a single modern urban-industrial society to match its adequate representation of societies with hunting and gathering, fishing, pastoral, and agricultural economies, thereby discriminating against the products of sociological as well as historical scholarship. I have consciously sought to avoid such disciplinary biases and to assure that the sample covers the widest possible range of known and adequately described cultures. That I have not wholly succeeded, however, is suggested by the apparent underrepresentation of societies with theories of the natural causation of illness, which could presumably have been corrected by including perhaps two additional societies from the modern urban-industrial world.

Coding

A crucial step in any cross-cultural research is to assess the societies of the sample for evidence on the presence, absence, and relative local importanc of the defined categories of data. This is called coding since the information is ordinarily entered in shorthand symbolic form on code sheets to facilitate comparisons. The coded data produced in this study have been presented in Tables 1 and 2. The ethnographic sources assessed are listed in the appendix.

The analysis was conducted by a corps of highly competent and experienced coders, all of whom had previously participated in comparable research and had full command of at least one major language other than English. Although the coding of sources in some of the less familiar foreign languages was done by other coders, the bulk of the work fell to Suzanne Frayser Wilson and Violetta Frederick. These two worked closely with each other and with me in the earlier phases of the research and rendered such valuable substantive as well as technical assistance that they were recognized as coauthors in the publication of the preliminary results of the study (Murdock, Wilson, and Frederick 1978).

When I disagreed with the coders over the interpretation of the evidence, they were usually able to convince me of the correctness of their judgments. For example, I noted a disturbing number of discrepancies between a paper on the evil eye by John Roberts (1976) and the codes produced for this study. When brought to the attention of Dr. Wilson, a number of the differences were found to be clearly the result of the fact that Roberts was interested in the evil eye as an example of what he calls "expressive culture" whereas our concern related solely to its use by witches as a technique for causing illness. Other seeming discrepancies merely reflect differences in definition, notably in the following cases: Among the Wolof (#21) the evil eye may cause a bride to lose her "purity," but there is no mention of its causing illness. Among the Wodaabe Fulani (#25) and the Maria Gond (#60) there is evidence that the evil eye may cause illness in cattle but not that it can have a similar effect on human beings. Among the Samoyed (#53), Orokaiva (#92), and Quiche (#155) the evil eye is or may be a technique of sorcery, but witchcraft as we have defined it is unknown. Among the Mbau Fijians (#102) the evil eye is reported as a technique by which aggressive spirits are believed to cause harm, but it is not a technique of either sorcery or witchcraft. For the Micmac (#126) the early sources make no mention of the evil eye, which does not appear in the ethnographic literature until centuries after the pinpointed date, when it had presumably been borrowed from the French Canadians.

In the cases of the Mbuti (#13), Mongo (#14), Tiv (#16), Hausa (#26), Lapps (#52), Tanala (#81), Ingalik (#122), Twana (#133), Klamath (#138), Chiricahua (#148), and Warrau (#162), the coders, in reviewing their decisions, were convinced of the greater accuracy of their own judgments, and this is confirmed by the fact that in none of these instances did Roberts have sufficient confidence in his own codes to label the evil eye as either "incontrovertibly present" (or absent) or "almost certainly present" (or absent). Only in the case of the Babylonians (#45) did I reject the judgment of the coders and accept that of Roberts. I did so on the basis of a personal communication from Samuel N. Kramer of the University of Pennsylvania, noted authority on early Mesopotamia, who confirmed the prevalence of both witchcraft and the evil eye in Babylonia at the time of Hammurabi and acknowledged personal acquaintance with cuneiform tablets prescribing formulas for obviating the baleful effects of the latter. In Chapter XI we shall encounter two more cases where it was found necessary to alter a code on the basis of additional information. On the whole, however, the coding appears to have been as accurate as it was meticulous.

Statistics

What distinguishes modern comparative research from earlier efforts is the abandonment of the previous procedure of analyzing masses of analogous "cases" torn from their cultural contexts and focusing of attention instead on "adhesions," that is, the extent to which traits coexist in the same cultures. When traits occur together, the possibility exists that they have influenced one another or become integrated, an unlikely eventuality if they occur only in different groups or at different times. This is, incidentally, the reason for the careful spatial and temporal pinpointing of the source materials in the appendix. Establishing tendencies to coexist requires statistical computations, and Tylor used a crude statistical technique in the same seminal paper (Tylor 1889) in which he proposed and illustrated the search for adhesions.

Decades elapsed before Tylor's innovation was taken up by a team consisting of a philosopher, an anthropologist, and a sociologist (Hobhouse, Wheeler, and Ginsberg 1915) in an ambitious undertaking flawed somewhat by carelessness. Next to accept Tylor's challenge, I produced first a trial paper (Murdock 1937) and then a major work (Murdock 1949) in which I applied the new procedure to the analysis of kinship and social organization. Not being trained in statistics, I have always sought and followed the advice of experts.

In this study all statistical data are presented in fourfold tables in which both the independent (row) and dependent (column) variables are dichotomized, for example, as present or absent, as important or unimportant, or as belonging or not to a particular category. In each correlation the null hypothesis, calculated in every case according to Fischer's Exact Test, measures the probability of the absence of a relationship, or tendency, in the data presented in the table. Total absence of any relationship would be indicated, for example, by a probability (p) of .5, but whenever p falls between .15 and .5 the significance level is considered too low for statistical validity.

Since none of the correlation coefficients in common use, such as gamma or Pearson's r, was adjudged adequate to measure the strengths of the various types of relationships revealed in the tables, it was decided to adopt an innovative alternative based on a proposal by Douglas R. White (1979), in which each table is classified by the logical type of its predominant relationship under one of a number of distinct tendencies. The format of the tables is illustrated in Correlation 1, which tests a distributional hypothesis concerniing the evil eye suggested by Roberts (1976). The four tendencies encountered in our correlations are defined as follows.

Tendency A occurs when the value of the cell on the upper right of a fourfold table is appreciably smaller than those of the other three cells. It indicates, technically speaking, that the presence of the independent (or row) variable tends to be a sufficient condition for the occurrence of the dependent (or column) variable. The strength of the tendency is measured by the percentage of the total number of cases which occur in the remaining three cells.

Correlation 1
Evil Eye as a Witchcraft Technique with the Circum-Mediterranean Region

	Evil Eye Reported as a Witchcraft Technique	Evil Eye as a Witchcraft Technique Absent or Unreported
Circum-Mediterranean Region	23	3
Other Ideological Regions	15	98

Null hypothesis: $p = .000000000003$
Tendency A: strength 98%

Tendency B occurs when the value of the cell on the lower left is appreciably smaller than those of the other three cells. It indicates that the presence of the independent variable tends to be a necessary (rather than sufficient) condition for the occurrence of the dependent variable. The strength of the tendency is measured by the percentage of cases which occur in the remaining three cells.

Tendency C occurs when the value of the cell on the upper left is appreciably smaller than those of the other three cells. It indicates that the presence of the independent variable tends to be a sufficient condition for the absence of the dependent variable (or that the occurrences of the independent and dependent variables tend to be mutually exclusive). The strength of the tendency is measured by the percentage of cases which occur in the remaining three cells.

Tendency D occurs when the value of the cell on the lower right is appreciably smaller than those of the other three cells. This indicates that the presence of the independent variable tends to be a necessary condition for the absence of the dependent variable (or that the combined occurrence of the independent and dependent variables tends to be exhaustive of the population sampled). The strength of the tendency is measured by the percentage of cases which occur in the remaining three cells.

I realize that statistics are distasteful to many otherwise informed people. I nevertheless urge the reader to make an effort to comprehend the method, at least approximately, for otherwise he will miss the flavor of some rather extraordinary findings.

Note

1. All these studies but Roberts 1976 are collected, along with other cross-cultural articles from *Ethnology,* in Herbert Barry III and Alice Schlegel, eds., *Cross-Cultural Samples and Codes* (Pittsburgh, 1980).

References Cited

Boas, F. The Limitations of the Comparative Method of Anthropology. Science, n.s., 4, 901–907. 1896.

Hobhouse, L. T., G. B. Wheeler, and M. Ginsberg. The Material Culture and Social Institutions of the Simpler Peoples. London, 1915.

Lagacé, R. O., ed. Sixty Cultures: A Guide to the HRAF Probability Sample Files. New Haven, 1977.

Murdock, G. P. Correlations of Matrilineal and Patrilineal Institutions. Studies in the Science of Society, ed. G. P. Murdock, pp. 445–470. New Haven, 1937.

———. Social Structure. New York, 1949.

———. Anthropology's Mythology. Proceedings of the Royal Anthropological Institute of Great Britain and Ireland for 1971, pp. 17–24. London, 1971.

Murdock, G. P., and D. R. White. Standard Cross-Cultural Sample. Ethnology 8: 329–369. 1969.

Murdock, G. P., S. F. Wilson, and V. Frederick. World Distribution of Theories of Illness. Ethnology 17: 449–470. 1978.

Roberts, J. M. Belief in the Evil Eye in World Perspective. The Evil Eye, ed. C. Moloney, pp. 223–278. New York, 1976.

Steward, J. H. Theory of Culture Change. Urbana, 1955.

Tylor, E. B. On a Method of Investigating the Development of Institutions. Journal of the Royal Anthropological Institute 18: 245–269. 1889.

White, D. R. Multivariate Entailment Analysis. Classifying Social Data, ed. H. C. Hudson. San Francisco, 1979.

V

Regional Analysis

The data on the typology of theories of illness were first ordered in terms of an impressionistic classification of the world's peoples in six ad hoc geographical regions which I had devised a decade ago. My object had been to divide the earth into regions with approximately equal areas and equal numbers of distinct peoples and cultures, so that the selection of roughly the same number of societies from each would produce a first approximation to a representative world sample for the statistical testing of cross-cultural hypotheses. North America, South America, and Oceania (with its continent of Australia and its many groups of islands from Indonesia to Polynesia) constituted readily distinguishable regions of comparable size and composition, but Africa and Asia were too large and Europe far too small. Trial and error showed, however, that if North Africa were detached from sub-Saharan Africa and the Near East from Asia, and if both were grouped with Europe to form a composite Circum-Mediterranean region, this would yield three regions reasonably comparable not only to one another but also to each American continent and the Insular Pacific.

The experimental tabulation of the incidence of the major theories of illness in these ad hoc regions led to a serendipitous discovery: The theories actually showed some tendency toward segregation by region. In particular, a disproportionate number of societies emphasizing witchcraft theories were found in Africa and the Circum-Mediterranean, of those stressing spirit aggression theories in East Asia and the Insular Pacific, and of those with preponderant sorcery theories in North and South America. In short, each of these pairs of regions revealed certain of the characteristics of culture areas, with tendencies toward both internal homogeneity and external differentiation. The reasons, however, were obscure, especially since culture areas are now recognized as strictly empirical rather than explanatory constructs.

It nevertheless seemed probable that the kinds of geographical criteria which had proved useful in delineating culture areas, particularly in North America, should be relevant in some manner to the differentiation of our impressionistic regions. Ocean barriers, for example, set limits to cultural diffusion and as a consequence often serve as boundaries of regions as well as of areas. However, careful analysis demonstrated that none of the most widely recognized geographic boundaries coincided with transitions from one to another type of ideational data: not the Sahara Desert, not the Himalaya Mountains, not Wallace's Line, nor the Bering Strait, nor the Isthmus of Panama. Invariably a few societies on one side of such a line showed stronger resemblances to the majority on the other side. Some qualification or supplementation of geographical criteria is obviously needed.

One obtrusive candidate is the criterion of race, in view of the well-known concentrations of Negroids in sub-Saharan Africa; of Caucasoids in the Circum-Mediterranean region; of Mongoloids in East Asia; of the Australoid, Papuan, Melanesian, Micronesian, and Polynesian subraces in the Insular Pacific; and of Amerindians in the New World. However, even apart from the extremely dubious propriety of applying biological criteria to cultural—and perhaps especially ideological—data, there are too many contradictory facts. None of the boundaries between the ad hoc regions coincides closely with racial borders, and in Africa the discrepancies are particularly striking. Such correspondences as do occur are almost certainly to be ascribed to certain basic similarities between (1) the factors that either segregate gene pools to produce both speciation and racial differentiation or else disperse them and (2) those which either inhibit or encourage cultural diffusion.

A second serendipitous discovery drew attention to the criterion of linguistic affiliation. We found that the prevalent theories of illness tend strongly to remain constant among the societies belonging to a particularly linguistic family. This is notably true of some of the largest groupings of linguistically cognate peoples in the world: (1) the speakers of Malayo-Polynesian, who dominate the Insular Pacific but also extend into continental southeast Asia; (2) the speakers of Indo-European, who predominate in Europe but extend eastward into India; and (3) the speakers of Afroasiatic or Hamito-Semitic, who dominate the Near East and North Africa but whose Chadic and Cushitic branches penetrate southward deep into Negro territory.

What is peculiarly characteristic of speech is that only mutually intelligible languages intergrade with one another in transitional zones as do racial and cultural differences. Otherwise the boundaries between linguistic groupings, including language families and sub-families, are invariably sharp. There are no truly intermediate or mixed languages; attempts to institute such concepts as Semi-Bantu and Nilo-Hamitic have invariably proved abortive. Language boundaries are barriers to communication and cultural diffusion, the more so the less mutually intelligible are the languages in question. Linguistic differences often aggravate political conflict, as between anglophones and francophones in Canada, the Croats and Serbs in Yugoslavia, and the Afrikanders and English speakers in South Africa. If language boundaries inhibit communication and foster divergent development, their absence promotes accommodation and syncretism. Moreover, these processes tend to persist over very long periods of time, barring major political upheavals or mass movements of population. David Olmsted (1957), for example, estimates by glottochronological tests that about three thousand years have passed since the ancestors of the diverse Bantu peoples of Africa formed a single speech community. And the Bantu as a whole form only one of seven branches of the Macro-Bantu subdivision of the Bantoid subfamily (or Central branch) of the Niger-Congo linguistic stock (Greenberg

1949). Additional millennia are required for divergence at each successive level in this developmental chain. Since linguistic boundaries are not only relatively easy to establish but extraordinarily stable over time, they are admirably suited for clarifying, supplementing, or refining cultural borders established by other criteria.

It was, therefore, decided to convert the ad hoc geographical regions, which had been based on nothing more than moderately informed guesswork, into what may be termed "ideational regions" by shifting the boundaries between them to accord more closely with the actual prevalence of the four major supernatural theories of illness—spirit aggression, sorcery, mystical retribution, and witchcraft—and at the same time to follow, insofar as possible, the borders between linguistic phyla. The reconstituted regions, still six in number after some relatively modest changes, may be appropriately defined in terms of the membership of their component societies in particular linguistic families and phyla. The identifying numbers of the individual societies are those listed in the Appendix and in Tables 1 and 2 in Chapters II and III.

The core of the reconstituted region of sub-Saharan Africa consists of the eighteen societies of the sample who speak languages of the Niger-Congo linguistic phylum: Thonga (#3) Mbundu (#5), Suku (#6), Nyakusa (#8), Chagga (#11a), Ganda (#12), Mongo (#14), Banen (#15), Tiv (#16), Fon (#18), Ashanti (#19), Mende (#20), Wolof (#21), Tallensi (#23), Fulani (#25), Massa (#27), Azande (#28), and Otoro (#30). With them are included three societies of the Khoisan phylum—the Nama Hottentot (#1), Kung Bushmen (#2), and Hadza (#9)—and two societies which reflect highly specialized historical circumstances: the Mbuti Pygmies (#13) and the Tanala (#81).

The Mbuti, like all the other members of the Pygmoid subrace, have been inundated for two thousand years by Negroid invaders with whom they have developed a dependent symbiotic relationship. The Pygmies have distinctively African cultures, but they have lost their original languages and have adopted those of the locally dominant Negro tribe, which in most cases is Bantu but is Central Sudanic in the special case of the Mbuti.

The Tanala, like other Malagasy peoples, are descended from Mongoloids who migrated from Indonesia nearly two thousand years ago to Madagascar by way of coastal East Africa. They still retain their Malayo-Polynesian language but are racially mixed with Caucasoids from Arabia and especially a heavy infusion of Negroid genes from imported African slaves. In culture their economy is African and their social organization basically Indonesian.

The core of the Circum-Mediterranean ideological region consists of the peoples of three large linguistic phyla, the Afroasiatic, Indo-Europen and Macro-Sudanic. The Afroasiatic phylum is represented by the Hausa (#26), Kaffa (#33), Somali (#36), Amhara (#37), Taureg (#41), Riffians (#42), Egyptians (#43), Hebrews (#44), Babylonians (#45), and Rwala Bedouin (#46); the Indo-European by the Gheg Albanians (#48), Romans (#49), Scots (#51a), Kurd (#57), and Uttar Pradesh (#63); the Macro-Sudanic by the Shilluk (#31), Dorobo (#34a), and Kenuzi Nubians (#39). The Macro-Sudanic peoples, who occupy territory extending southward from Nubia in Egypt to the Masai in northern Tanzania, are remarkable because, although unmistakably Negroid in physique, they affiliate more strongly in the ideology of illness with the Caucasoid peoples to the north than with their racial kinsmen to the south. Also included in the Circum-Mediterranean region, on ideological as well as geographic bounds, are the Basques (#50) of Europe, the Gond (#60) and Toda (#61) of the Dravidian family in India, and three societies with isolated languages on the fringes of the Sahara: the Songhai (#24), Mao (#32), and Teda (#40). Likewise grouped here are two societies of the Turkic family of the Altaic linguistic phylum— the Turks (#47) and Kazak (#65). These are noteworthy as representing the only instance where our criteria have compelled us to split peoples with cognate languages between two ideological regions, since representatives of the Mongolic and Tungusic families of the Altaic phylum are assigned to East Asia.

The East Asian ideological region is composed of the speakers of numerous relatively small linguistic families: the Lapps (#52) and Samoyed (#53) of the Uralic family; the Mongols (#66) and Manchu (#115) of the Altaic phylum; the Lepcha (#68), Garo (#69), and Burmese (#71) of the Sino-Tibetan phylum; the Lamet (#72), Semang (#77), and Nicobarese (#78) of the Mon-Khmer family; the Aleut (#123) and Copper Eskimo (#124) of the Eskimauan family; and the independent families represented by the Vietnamese (#73), Siamese (#76), Andamanese (#79), Japanese (#117), Ainu (#118), Yukaghir (#120), and Chukchee (#121).

In addition to the more populous societies of eastern and southeastern Asia, the East Asia region embraces the vast expanse of the so-called Circumpolar peoples and cultures from the Lapps in northern Europe to the Angmagsalik Eskimo in eastern Greenland—a span of more than three hundred degrees longitude or five-sixths of the circumference of the earth. The boundary with the North American region is that between the speakers of Eskimauan languages to the west and north and those of Athapaskan and Algonkian to the south and east.

The Insular Pacific ideological region is dominated by speakers of the far-flung Malayo-Polynesian or Austronesian linguistic phylum, whose twenty representatives in our sample extend from the Rhade (#74) of Indo-China and the Atayal (#113) of Formosa to Easter Island in the remote Pacific. With them are included on geographical grounds two tribes of the Australian family—the Tiwi (#90) and Aranda (#91)—and three of the Papuan phylum—the Orokaiva (#92), Kapauku (#94), and Siuai (#99).

Both the North American and South American ideological regions are composed of peoples of many diverse linguistic families. North America includes all of the societies in Tables 1 and 2 from the Ingalik (#122) of Alaska to the Quiche (#155) of Guatemala, and

South America all those from the Miskito (#156) of Honduras to
the Yahgan (#186) of Tierra del Fuego. Among the latter are two
transplanted Negro societies—the Haitians (#160) and Saramacca
(#165)—who merit special notice.

The Haitians of the Caribbean are descended from imported Negro
slaves with negligible Caucasoid and Amerindian admixture. They
speak a dialect of French, the Indo-European language of Haiti's
colonial conquerors, with a strong infusion of Niger-Congo loan
words. Their culture, too, is mixed European and African.

The Saramacca of Surinam are a "Bush Negro" people descended
from slaves who escaped from their European masters into the "bush,"
where they lived in close proximity to the indigenous Amerindian
tribes but in time achieved essential political autonomy. Though they
are basically Negroid in race, their culture shows strong affinities with
those of the neighboring Guiana Indians. Their language is reported
to be "pidginized" Indo-European with strong Niger-Congo ingredi-
ents and numerous Amerindian loan words.

Table 3 (Table 2 in Murdock et al. 1978) presents summary and
supplementary information pertinent to the following characteriza-
tion of the reconstructed ideational regions.

Africa ranks very high in theories of mystical retribution, which are
reported for all but one of its societies and are important (i.e., either
predominant or significant) in half of them. Violations of sex and
etiquette taboos are more common as precipitating factors than in any
other region. Spirit aggression and sorcery are also prevalent theories,
and of about equal importance. Africa uses the techniques of contagious magic to cause illness more frequently than do other regions,
but the otherwise widespread sorcery technique of spirit possession is
very rare. Ancestors are more common as supernatural aggressors
than in other regions. Witchcraft is important among about a third
of Africa's peoples but is absent in about half of them, and there are
only sporadic reports of belief in the evil eye, mainly on the northern
fringe of the region.

The *Circum-Mediterranean* shows an enormously higher incidence of witchcraft theories than any other region. They are reported for every society except the remote Maria Gond (#60) of India and are an important cause of illness in 62 percent of them. In striking confirmation of the findings of John Roberts, the technique of the evil eye is attested for 88 percent of the societies in the region. Witchcraft is nevertheless outranked by spirit aggression, which rates as important in 96 percent of the constituent societies. Supernatural aggressors are more commonly major deities or gods than elsewhere in the world. The region ranks low in theories of sorcery, and even lower in those of mystical retribution with the fewest relevant taboos and a rating of important for only 8 percent of its societies.

East Asia is noteworthy for its unanimous acceptance of the theory of spirit aggression, which is reported for 100 percent of its component societies and ranks as either the predominant theory or as an important secondary one in all of them. The alleged aggressors are spirits or demons more frequently than elsewhere in the world. The region ranks lowest of all in the incidence of sorcery theories and almost as low in those of mystical retribution. Witchcraft theories, so important in the two regions to the west, are virtually absent here and in the three regions farther east.

The *Insular Pacific* likewise ranks high in theories of spirit aggression, which are reported for all of its societies and are important in 92 percent of them. The region also reveals a high incidence of sorcery theories, which are reported for all but one of its component societies and are important in more than half. Among sorcery techniques, those of verbal spells and exuvial magic have their strongest representation in this region. Theories of mystical retribution reveal an incidence slightly below average despite the popular reputation of Polynesia for the number and variety of its taboos.

North America outranks all other regions in theories of sorcery, which occur in all of its societies without exception and are reported as important in 83 percent of them. Among its techniques, object intrusion and presumptive poison appear more frequently than in any

Table 3
Regional Distribution of Theories of Illness, with Ratings

Categories and Ratings	Sub-Saharan Africa	Circum-Mediterranean	East Asia	Insular Pacific	North America	South America
			Number of Societies in			
Total	23	26	19	25	24	22
Spirit aggression ratings						
Predominant	7	13	17	20	9	12
Significant	9	12	2	3	6	8
Minor	6	1	0	2	8	2
Absent	1	0	0	0	1	0
Sorcery ratings						
Predominant	1	1	0	5	11	10
Significant	12	5	5	8	9	5
Minor	8	13	10	11	4	4
Absent	2	7	4	1	0	3
Sorcery techniques						
Contagious magic	11	3	4	10	2	4
Exuvial magic	5	6	4	7	6	4
Imitative magic	1	7	5	7	5	5
Object intrusion	3	0	2	4	17	11
Presumptive poison	6	2	3	3	8	7
Spirit possession	1	3	5	7	3	7
Soul theft	1	0	3	3	3	6
Verbal spells	8	9	5	15	6	4

Mystical retribution ratings						
Predominant	4	0	0	0	1	0
Significant	7	2	4	9	10	2
Minor	11	10	11	12	12	15
Absent	1	14	4	4	1	5
Sinful taboo violations						
Etiquette taboos	10	4	4	4	5	2
Food taboos	12	6	8	12	17	11
Ritual taboos	4	2	5	8	9	1
Sex taboos	12	6	5	8	3	9
Sensory taboos	7	5	9	10	16	9
Witchcraft ratings						
Predominant	4	5	0	0	0	0
Significant	4	11	0	1	2	0
Minor	2	9	3	3	5	5
Absent	13	1	16	21	17	17
Witchcraft techniques						
Evil eye	5	23	1	2	4	3
Other techniques only	5	2	2	2	3	2

other region. With regard to theories of mystical retribution, North America shares the lead with Africa but ranks first in food, ritual, and sensory taboos. By contrast, it ranks at the very bottom in theories of spirit aggression, which are absent or of only minor importance in more than one third of its societies.

South America, on the other hand, ranks high in theories of spirit aggression, which are recorded as present in 100 percent of its societies and as important in 91 percent of them. Ghosts appear as supernatural aggressors more frequently than in other regions. The continent ranks next to North America in theories of sorcery and as the highest of all regions in the techniques of soul theft and spirit aggression. It shows an extremely low incidence of theories of mystical retribution, which are reported as important for only two of its societies.

The distributional evidence on theories of illness poses a variety of fundamental scientific problems, including: (1) Why do theories of illness that totally lack scientific respectability receive so much more widespread recognition than theories that medical science is ready to accept? (2) Why are four particular types of supernatural theories (those of spirit aggression, sorcery, mystical retribution, and witchcraft) preferred so strikingly to the others? (3) What accounts for the widely varying incidence of the four, ranging from near universality for one of them (spirit aggression theories), through sporadic and irregular occurrence for two of them, to essential confinement to a single region for one of them (witchcraft theories)?

References Cited

Greenberg, J. H. Studies in African Linguistic Classification. Southwestern Journal of Anthropology 5: 309–317. 1949.

Murdock, G. P., S. F. Wilson, and V. Frederick. World Distribution of Theories of Illness. Ethnology 17: 449–470. 1978.

Olmsted, D. L. Three Tests of Glottochronological Theory. American Anthropologist 59: 834–842. 1957.

VI

Man's Ideational Environment

There is probably heuristic value in analyzing the world in which man lives and functions into three components: his physical environment, his social environment, and his ideational environment. The first, consisting of the material aspects of external reality, and the second, consisting of the groups and categories of human beings with whom individuals interact, are real in the sense that they form the context that determines which of man's reactions will encounter success and be perpetuated, that is, in technical terms, which will be positively reinforced. (My psychological orientation is approximately that of Miller and Dollard [1941]).

It is important to note, however, that success reinforces all the responses in a given set or series regardless of whether they have actually contributed to that success or are, so to speak, parasitic. Prominent among the parasitic items in man's technological responses to his physical environment are the rites of hunting magic and garden magic that proliferate in ethnographic accounts of the food quest. They are perpetuated because of the effectiveness of the associated productive techniques of hunting and tillage and are eliminated only as technology is gradually converted through systematic experimentation into science. The relationship between magic and science was dimly recognized by Sir James Frazer when he characterized the former as false science. Actually, of course, magic is illusory technology whereas science is the most admirable component of man's ideational environment.

53

In theory the principle of reinforcement should operate in the social as in the physical environment, and few would question that social behavior can be either adaptive or maladaptive. There are innumerable manuals setting forth rules of etiquette and prescriptions for making friends and influencing people, the most famous of which is probably Machiavelli's advice to princes on how to govern effectively. Other people can be cajoled, beguiled, tempted, admonished, bribed, bamboozled, coerced, or otherwise persuaded to alter their behavior by so wide a variety of techniques in such an infinitude of combinations that even such experts at persuasion as politicians, advertisers, and clergymen would be at a loss to calculate them. As a result of this state of confusion, the reinforcement principle has proved incapable of effectively segregating the valid from the parasitic in the ideology of social behavior, and virtually undisciplined imagination has held sway. The resulting ideologies, to be sure, give clear evidence of their origins since they consist largely, not of magical notions originating from technology, but of concepts of supernatural beings derived from a human model.

These products of the human imagination, however fascinating, do not, at least to me, evoke a degree of admiration comparable to that inspired by a parallel component of the ideational environment, the highly generalized and streamlined codes of ethics propounded by such world figures as Confucius and Jesus.

It is perhaps unnecessary to insist that, unlike the physical and social environments, the ideational environment is totally illusory and has no actual existence outside of peoples' minds. There are, for example, no such things as souls, spirits, or demons, and such mental constructs as Jehovah are as fictitious as are those of Superman or Santa Claus. Neither ghosts nor gods exert the slightest influence on men or their behavior. But men can and do influence the behavior of one another, and the ideas they hold can have a serious bearing on how they behave. The Crusades, the Inquisition, and Hitler's "holocaust" illustrate, not strictly the power of ideas, but the influence that can be exerted by men who hold particular ideas.

Theories of illness constitute a significant part of the ideational environment. Those of natural causation require no explanation other than their presumed validity. On the other hand, the theories of supernatural causation, which would easily be recognized as parasitic if they were not numerically so preponderant, need to be accounted for. This is not an anthropological problem despite our use of ethnographic data; it is a general behavioral science problem. As such, its solution must necessarily accord with the basic principles of behavioral psychology, as George Homans (1967) has so insightfully pointed out.

The psychological mechanism of projection figures prominently in my interpretations. In this respect I follow in the footsteps of Whiting and Child (1953), who were the first to apply the concept of projection effectively in dealing with theories of illness. My basic theoretical orientation differs only slightly, though perhaps significantly, from theirs. The position of Whiting and Child is that differences in child-training practices generate deeply rooted habitual response tendencies and that these persist into later life when they give rise, through projection, to one or another of the theories of illness. The present volume assumes, however, that it is not alone the experience of the individual undergoing socialization in infancy and childhood that is relevant, but his total experience with social control on into adulthood. It is this total experience that provides the source of the projections which generate and maintain fundamental ideological concepts such as theories of illness.

If the assumption of Whiting and Child were valid, one would expect considerably more diversity than actually occurs among the societies of a region and considerably less average difference between regions. Specific illustrations, however, may prove more convincing. On our shared assumption that techniques of sorcery arise through the mechanism of projection, those of object intrusion would seem to reflect the experience of adult males in propelling arrows with bows, darts with blowguns, or javelins with spear-throwers. The technique of presumptive poison similarly suggests projection from the experience of adult females in foraging for roots, berries, and fruits and in distinguishing the edible from the poisonous. The technique of verbal spells would seem to presuppose persons of either sex sufficiently mature to have attained full mastery of the indigenous language. Moreover, the custodians and arbiters of supernatural beliefs and practices in nearly all societies are the adult men and/or women who function as shamans.

References Cited

Homans, G. C. The Nature of Social Science. New York, 1967.
Miller, N. E., and J. Dollard. Social Learning and Imitation. New Haven, 1941.
Whiting, J. W. M., and I. L. Child. Child Training and Personality. New Haven, 1953.

VII

Witchcraft Theories
and the Circum-Mediterranean

Witchcraft is a concern of this study only to the extent that it is believed to cause illness in human beings. Such notions as witches transporting themselves through the air on broomsticks or forgathering on Walpurgis Night or mischievously causing the milk of dairy cows to dry up are considered irrelevant and were ignored by coders in the absence of specific evidence of their presumed capacity and propensity for causing illness in other people. For an understanding of witchcraft in general the reader should look elsewhere, for example, in such well-regarded works as Evans-Pritchard (1937) and Kluckhohn (1942).

Witchcraft theories differ sharply in their geographical distribution from all other theories of illness, natural or supernatural. They are concentrated in a core area of contiguous societies, taper off at its margins, and occur only rarely and sporadically outside of its limits—a pattern reminiscent of the culture areas established for North America by Wissler (1917) and Kroeber (1939). The core area is practically coextensive with the Circum-Mediterranean ideological region, although it does not include the remote Maria Gond (#60) of central India and in the south spills over into adjacent Africa to include such peoples as the Banen (#15), Tiv (#16), Ashanti (#19), Wolof (#21), and Azande (#28).

Culture areas were constructed to account for the distribution not of single traits but of trait complexes composed of a number of elements either functionally related, like the saddle, bridle, stirrups, picket lines, and corrals in the horse complex of the Plains Indians, or assembled through the accidents of history. Witchcraft theories can readily be viewed as belonging to a trait complex which also includes ideas about the techniques employed by witches and the counter-measures taken by their victims. Prominent among these is the concept of the evil eye and the practices associated therewith, which are documented in an encyclopedic work by Seligmann (1910) and which Correlation 1 has already demonstrated to be closely associated with the Circum-Mediterranean.

Culture area theorists have commonly speculated that trait complexes are likely to have originated at a culture center in or near the heart of the core area. In this connection it may be relevant to note that Mesopotamia is located at the approximate geographical center of the Circum-Mediterranean region and that beliefs in witchcraft, the evil eye, and protective formulas against the latter are attested in cuneiform tablets for the Babylonians by at least the time of Hammurabi around 1750 B.C.

Also characteristic of a culture area are the generally decreasing importance of beliefs in witchcraft causation and the increasing variability in such associated traits as the evil eye along the margins of the Circum-Mediterranean core area. Moreover, a substantial portion of the scattered occurrences of witchcraft theories outside the Circum-Mediterranean region are reported for societies that have been conquered or colonized by peoples from the core area, for example, the Spaniards, from whom they are quite likely to have borrowed the complex. In short, there are some fairly substantial grounds for regarding the Circum-Mediterranean as a culture area in which one of the most characteristic and deep-seated traits is the belief in the causation of illness by witchcraft.

Distributional and historical evidence for other Circum-Mediterranean cultural phenomena seems to lead to parallel conclusions. Writing, for instance, appears to have been first invented in ancient Sumer, reinvented (perhaps by stimulus diffusion) in early Egypt, improved by the Phoenicians, Arabs, Greeks, and Romans, and spread throughout most of the Circum-Mediterranean and beyond, with independent inventions in China and Mexico. Since its history thus roughly parallels that of witchcraft theories and the evil eye, writing should reveal a similar regional distribution. This is corroborated in Correlation 2, which intercorrelates our data with the code on writing and records in Murdock and Provost (1973).

Correlation 2

Use of True Writing with the Circum-Mediterranean Region

	A System of True Writing in Use	No System of Writing in Use
Circum-Mediterranean region	18	8
Other ideological regions	13	100

Null hypothesis: $p = .000000007$
Tendency A: strength 94%

Influenced by Guy Swanson's stimulating book *The Birth of the Gods* (1960), I coded evidence on the presence or absence of a belief in a high god and the degree of his presumable concern with human affairs in Column 34 of the *Ethnographic Atlas* (Murdock 1967). The great majority of the world's societies that exhibit such beliefs have accepted or been influenced by one or more of three great religions that originated among and spread primarily to the peoples of the Circum-Mediterranean region, namely Judaism, Christianity, and Islam. Intercorrelation with the coded data of the present study should therefore reveal a regional correlation similar to the previous one. Correlation 3 provides the proof.

These cultural traits which correlate so spectacularly with the Circum-Mediterranean region would, of course, reveal comparable correlations with one another and with other traits having similar historical associations. This might have satisfied Franz Boas and his historically minded colleagues who dominated the American scene

Correlation 3
Belief in a Concerned High God with the Circum-Mediterranean Region

	A High God Believed Present and Concerned with Human Affairs	A High God Lacking or Considered Otiose
Circum-Mediterranean region	18	8
Other ideological regions	21	78

Null hypothesis: p = .0000075
Tendency A: strength 94%

fifty years ago when I was just embarking on my professional career in anthropology, but they satisfy few scholars today. The drawing of historical inferences from geographical distributions rests too heavily on oversimple conceptions of diffusion and tells too little about the acutal causes of change. Though superior to the elaborate verbal interpretations favored by philosophers and literary critics, they fall far short of a type acceptable to scientists, namely, those which establish probable functional or cause-and-effect relationships. Only two sophisticated methods of establishing such relationships are available —through experiment or through statistics—and of these only the latter is possible in the human sciences.

Even a plethora of regional or historical associations does not preclude the possibility of finding genuine functional associations for which the correlations are high and uncontaminated by obvious regional factors. A search of the sources presenting coded ethnographic material has produced two with pertinent data. Evidence on the presence of a patrilineal rule of descent (or of the closely related rule of double descent) as coded by Murdock and Wilson (1972), when juxtaposed with our own data on witchcraft theories of illness, yields Correlation 4. There are at least two reasons for this correlation. First, on account of its usual association with patrilocal residence,

Correlation 4
Witchcraft Theories of Illness with Patrilineal Descent

	Witchcraft Theories Important	Witchcraft Theories Absent or Unimportant
Patrilineal or double descent	21	43
Matrilineal, ambilineal, or bilateral descent	6	69

Null hypothesis: $p = .00022$
Tendency B: strength 96%

patrilineal descent tends to remove a married woman from her own close relatives and to place her in a social milieu of comparative strangers. Second, patrilineal descent is especially conducive to polygyny, so that a married woman is forced into close association with co-wives rather than sisters—a situation particularly likely to engender jealousy, envy, and spite, the characteristic emotional concomitants of witchcraft.

A second nonregional correlate of witchcraft theories of illness is the payment of a substantial bride-price in marriage as contrasted with other modes of contracting marriage. The comparative data for Correlation 5 were obtained from Column 12 of the *Ethnographic Atlas* (Murdock 1967). The underlying hypothesis is that payment of a bride-price in marriage creates invidious distinctions among women and arouses envy in men who are insufficiently endowed with material goods to compete successfully for the women they desire.

Correlation 5 supports the conclusion from Correlation 4 that conditions that tend to arouse envy and related emotions are also conducive to the development of witchcraft theories of illness. In addition to patrilineal descent and the payment of a bride-price as the customary mode of marriage, such conditions include the prevalence of marked differences in ascribed social statuses, as will be demonstrated

Correlation 5

Witchcraft Theories of Illness with Payment of a Bride-Price

	Witchcraft Theories Important	Witchcraft Theories Absent or Unimportant
Payment of a substantial bride-price in marriage	17	37
Any other mode of marriage in effect	10	73

Null hypothesis: p = .0054
Tendency B: strength 92%

in Correlation 10 (see Chapter VIII). But the presence of favorable conditions is not a sufficient explanation, for envy is presumably a universal human emotion whereas witchcraft theories of illness have essentially only a regional distribution. Some specific ideational connection between envy and the causation of illness is also needed.

Such a connection is supplied quite satisfactorily by the belief that illness can be caused by a glance of an envious person possessing the magical power of the evil eye. Unlike the emotion of envy, belief in the evil eye is not universal but has a regional distribution, as was demonstrated in Correlation 1. It is, then, the presumably accidental conjunction of a belief in witchcraft with the conception of the evil eye as a technique for causing illness that accounts for the essential confinement of the witchcraft theory of illness to the Circum-Mediterranean region and for its apparent membership in a localized trait complex.

References Cited

Evans-Pritchard, E. E. Witchcraft, Oracles and Magic among the Azande. Oxford, 1937.

Kluckhohn, C. Navaho Witchcraft. Papers of the Peabody Museum of American Archaeology and Ethnology, Harvard University 22: ii, 1–149. 1942.

Kroeber, A. L. Cultural and Natural Areas of Native North America. University of California Publications in American Archaeology and Ethnology 38: 1–242. 1939.

Murdock, G. P. Ethnographic Atlas. Pittsburgh, 1967.

Murdock, G. P., and C. Provost. Measurement of Cultural Complexity. Ethnology 12: 379–392. 1973.

Murdock, G. P., and S. F. Wilson. Settlement Patterns and Community Organization. Ethnology 12: 254–293. 1972.

Seligmann, S. Der böse Blick. 2 vols. Berlin, 1910.

Swanson, G. E. The Birth of the Gods. Ann Arbor, 1960.

Wissler, C. The American Indian. New York, 1917.

VIII

The Antithesis of Sorcery
and Witchcraft Theories

Superficially the theories of the causation of illness by sorcery and by witchcraft appear to be mere variants of a single cause—the malevolent use of magical techniques to injure another human being. Students and laymen invariably confuse them, and even professional anthropologists are not always clear about their distinction. Such mistakes are not surprising since few educated people have had any first-hand experience with either. Actually the two theories are unrelated and in most respects entirely antithetical to each other. The supporting evidence for this conclusion will be presented before the contrast itself is explicitly formulated.

In the first place, the occurrences of the two theories are negatively rather than positively correlated in the sample at large, as is established in Correlation 6. In other words, where one is present the other is likely to be absent—an improbable eventuality if both were dependent on the same or similar causal factors.

In the second place, sorcery and witchcraft theories tend to be associated with societies having contrasting levels of cultural complexity, the former with simpler or more primitive cultures, the latter with more advanced ones. This is demonstrated by their divergent correlations with the most widely recognized criterion of cultural complexity, the use of a system of true writing. Correlations 7 and 8 draw upon data from the codes in Murdock and Provost (1973). Of the two correlations, that with sorcery theories is negative whereas that with witchcraft theories is positive.

Correlation 6
Witchcraft Theories with Sorcery Theories of Illness

	Witchcraft Theories Important	Witchcraft Theories Absent or Unimportant
Sorcery theories important	8	64
Sorcery theories absent or unimportant	19	48

Null hypothesis: p = .009
Tendency C: strength 95%

Correlation 7
Sorcery Theories with the Use of True Writing

	Sorcery Theories Important	Sorcery Theories Absent or Unimportant
Societies with true writing	10	21
Preliterate societies	62	46

Null hypothesis: p = .01
Tendency C: strength 93%

In the third place, the two theories tend to cluster in different regions. Witchcraft theories, as was demonstrated in Chapter VII, are strongly associated with the Circum-Mediterranean region, whereas sorcery theories, as indicated in Correlation 9, preponderate in the New World.

The evidence of these correlations makes abundantly clear the fundamental antithesis between sorcery and witchcraft theories. The basis of the distinction is implicit in the definitions of the two theories. Sorcery can be employed by anyone—male or female, noble or com-

Correlation 8

Witchcraft Theories with the Use of True Writing

	Witchcraft Theories Important	Witchcraft Theories Absent or Unimportant
Societies with true writing	11	20
Preliterate societies	16	92

Null hypothesis: p = .01
Tendency C: strength 92%

Correlation 9

Sorcery Theories with the North and South American Regions

	Sorcery Theories Important	Sorcery Theories Absent or Unimportant
North and South America	35	11
Other ideological regions	37	56

Null hypothesis: p = .000045
Tendency A: strength 92%

moner—who commands the appropriate techniques. If a would-be sorcerer lacks knowledge of the right technique, he has the option of employing a specialist, a shaman, to perform the appropriate verbal spell or magical rite in his behalf. Sorcery techniques are, in short, a sort of ideological equivalent of technology, available for anyone who wants or needs them. Societies in which access to supernatural power is widely distributed among the population provide exceptionally fertile ground for the development of sorcery theories of illness. This is notably the case in western North America, where children of both sexes are dispatched repeatedly into the wilderness in a quest for guardian spirits who will provide them for life with a variety of valued supernatural powers and immunities.

A witch, in contrast to a person who resorts to sorcery, is "a member of a special class of human beings believed to be endowed with a special power and propensity for evil." His or her power is an intrinsic attribute, a sort of class prerogative, not an acquired skill accessible to anyone. The effects of sorcery can be offset by counter sorcery, for example, exorcism of an alien spirit or removal of an intrusive foreign object, but the major technique of witchcraft, the evil eye, leaves no traces and victims are forced to rely on such fallible protective devices as amulets and verbal formulas.

When witchcraft is suspected, attention is likely to be directed to any category of powerful or privileged persons, including the well-born, the wealthy, and those with political authority. Since these are usually secure, it tends to be deflected or displaced to other noticeable but unpopular types of people—foreigners, hunchbacks, senile women, or individuals with piercing stares.

From the foregoing it would seem logical to expect beliefs in witch-craft and theories of illness deriving therefrom to be positively corre-lated with complexity in social stratification. Correlation 10 tests and

Correlation 10

Witchcraft Theories of Illness with Social Classes

	Witchcraft Theories Important	Witchcraft Theories Absent or Unimportant
Societies with definite social classes or castes	16	32
Societies lacking class and caste distinctions	11	75

Null hypothesis: $p = .005$
Tendency B: strength 92%

verifies the association of witchcraft theories with the presence of definite social classes or castes as coded in Murdock and Provost (1973).

Money provides a medium by which one form of property can be converted into another or into services or even wives. Its availability in a society should therefore operate to accentuate status differences and hence to favor the development of witchcraft theories of illness. This hypothsis is corroborated in Correlation 11 with the aid of coded data from Murdock and Provost (1973).

Correlation 11

Witchcraft Theories with Money as a Medium of Exchange

	Witchcraft Theories Important	Witchcraft Theories Absent or Unimportant
Societies possessing true money	20	51
Societies lacking true money	7	61

Null hypothesis: $p = .0066$
Tendency B: strength 95%

The results of Correlation 11 are entirely consistent with the finding in Correlation 5 that witchcraft theories are also positively correlated with the payment of a substantial bride-price in marriage. Correlation 12 draws upon coded data in the *Ethnographic Atlas* (Murdock 1967) to make a parallel test of the association of sorcery theories with the practice of paying a bride-price. In this case the correlation turns out to be strongly negative rather than positive, and its magnitude is such as to give further dramatic emphasis to the antithesis between sorcery and witchcraft theories of illness.

The clinching contrast between witchcraft and sorcery, however, is seen in their differing relationship to magical therapy. Both are cited

Correlation 12

Sorcery Theories of Illness with Payment of a Bride-Price

	Sorcery Theories Important	Sorcery Theories Absent or Unimportant
Payment of a substantial bride-price in marriage	19	36
Any other mode of marriage in effect	53	31

Null hypothesis: $p = .0009$
Tendency C: strength 86%

with some frequency as causes of illness, but witchcraft is practically never reported as contributing in any way to its cure. The techniques of sorcery, on the other hand, almost universally provide a basis for magical therapy. An individual who controls the techniques for producing illness by magical means necessarily possesses knowledge that can be applied to counteract the efforts of other sorcerers. If he can cause illness, he can presumably help treat similar ailments. Such a person is a shaman, a combination of sorcerer and therapist, and to his kind a considerable portion of the peoples of the world entrust the bulk of the practice of medicine. He is, consequently, the medicine man par excellence.

A shaman must have a thorough knowledge of the ideology of sorcery as it is understood in his society in order to engage in magical therapy. But he need not practice it very often, if at all. There is abundant evidence that it is therapy rather than aggressive sorcery that has engaged the primary attention of medicine men the world over. A shaman does not require actual experience in the administration of presumptive poison to be able to prescribe a purgative for a victimized patient, or in the practice of exuvial magic if he knows enough to search for a concealed nail clipping or lock of the patient's hair. All he needs is the requisite knowledge and a reputation for the capacity to apply it successfully.

Sorcery is undoubtedly used for aggressive purposes, but most ethnographers believe that it is actually practiced much less frequently than it is suspected. I have evidence on this point from my fieldwork among the Tenino Indians in 1934–35, when I had the good fortune to secure the services as an informant of the most respected shaman in the tribe. After mutual confidence had been established on other topics, the subject of magical therapy was introduced. I aroused deep interest in the shaman by my knowledge of the beliefs and practices of other societies, and ultimately the two of us exchanged information with the zest of a pair of professional colleagues "talking shop." The shaman, who was well over eighty years of age and could remember life conditions prior to the establishment of the reservation, freely discussed the techniques of therapy that he had employed over the years. These were directed in the main toward the exorcism of animal spirits which had supposedly been dispatched by other shamans to take possession of the bodies of his patients. He ultimately admitted that on occasion he had also applied his knowledge aggressively, but he could recall only three such instances in his entire professional career. One of them was the unintended death of an innocent young girl, the recollection of which aroused in him unmistakable feelings of guilt. His other two victims were notorious malefactors who had exhausted the patience of the community and whose removal was considered a public service. (The Tenino lacked formal judicial procedures capable of dealing effectively with habitual antisocial behavior.)

The ethnographic literature leaves the impression that a very limited use of aggressive sorcery, as compared with magical therapy, is probably typical of shamanism elsewhere in the world. The medicine man in simple societies is primarily a healer rather than a sorcerer and is respected appreciably more than he is feared. Witches, however, are believed to use their powers for exclusively malign purposes, and they are consequently loathed as well as feared.

References Cited

Murdock, G. P. Ethnographic Atlas. Pittsburgh, 1967.

Murdock, G. P., and C. Provost. Measurement of Cultural Complexity. Ethnology 21: 379–392. 1973.

IX

Incidence of Spirit Aggression Theories

The most obtrusive fact about spirit aggression theories of illness is their virtual universality. When the coders completed their analysis, I observed that they had recorded the presence of such theories in 135 of the 139 societies of the sample and concluded that they were absent only among the Hadza (#9), Riffians (#42), Slave (#128), and Omaha (#143). This extraordinarily high incidence, coupled with the universality of overt human aggression and the seeming obviousness of its projection to supernatural beings, suggested the possibility that the four exceptional codings might represent either oversights on the part of the ethnographers or errors on the part of the coders and that spirit aggression theories of illness might possibly rank among the few genuine universals of human culture. It therefore seemed advisable to check the codes in question by seeking additional evidence.

For the Omaha I consulted a monograph by Reo Fortune (1932) which the coders had not examined and found the following statement on page 77: "Ghosts are greatly feared because they have powers of spirit abstraction from the living, so causing delirium, madness and unconsciousness, often leading to death." This obviously contradicted the negative conclusion of the coder, and the code was changed accordingly.

For the Riffians an inquiry addressed to their principal ethnographer, Carleton Coon, elicited the reply, "The Riffians attribute most of their ailments to Jinns," coupled with a reference to specific data in a recent monograph by David Hart (1976: 154–159). Clearly the coder was also in error in this case, and the Riffians cannot be counted as an exception to the postulated universality of theories of spirit aggression.

A similar inquiry was addressed to June Helm, the principal authority on the Slave. In her response she indicated that, though aware of the possibility, she had never actually encountered, either in her personal fieldwork or in the earlier literature, any indication that the Slave Indians ascribe illness to the direct agency of supernatural beings. Since all the other Athapaskan-speaking societies in our sample, including the nearby Kaska (#129), are reported to hold spirit aggression theories of illness, it is virtually certain that the ancestors of the Slave held similar views at some time in the past and have presumably abandoned them under some special set of local circumstances. A similar explanation may also apply to the Hadza, since the other Khoisan-speaking societies in the sample regard spirit aggression as the predominant cause of illness.

Nevertheless, it would be improper to reject the judgments of the coders on such speculative grounds. It seems preferable to conclude that spirit aggression theories are only quasi-universals rather than genuine cultural universals. This conclusion may, in fact, have a wider application. When I asserted in an earlier work (Murdock 1949: 2–13) the universality of certain features of social organization, notably marriage, the nuclear family, and primary incest taboos, I was widely charged with ignoring some very rare exceptions, such as the Israeli kibbutz. I am now prepared to admit that there may actually be no absolute cultural universals but only a limited number of peculiarly interesting cultural phenomena which occur everywhere except under highly exceptional sets of circumstances. Belief in spirit aggression as a cause of illness is conceivably such a quasi-universal.

Spirit aggression theories show no tendency to cluster in a particular ideational region as do witchcraft theories. Table 2 has revealed that they are rated as important (i.e., predominant or significant) in a majority of the societies in all six regions, most markedly so in East

Asia and the Circum-Mediterranean. Since these are the two regions with the highest average level of cultural complexity, it is not surprising that spirit aggression theories are positively correlated with a number of the indices of cultural complexity assembled in Murdock and Provost (1973). Correlation 13, for example, shows such a relationship between spirit aggression theories and the use of writing.

Correlation 13

Spirit Aggression Theories with the Use of Writing

	Spirit Aggression Theories Important	Spirit Aggression Theories Absent or Unreported
Societies with true writing	30	1
Preliterate societies	99	20

Null hypothesis: p = .026
Tendency A: strength 99%

The positive results in Correlation 13 are confirmed by those in Correlation 14, which employs the level of political integration as a measure of complexity. A petty state is defined as one with only a

Correlation 14

Spirit Aggression Theories with Complexity of Political Organization

	Spirit Aggression Theories Important	Spirit Aggression Theories Unimportant or Unreported
Societies with organized states of large or medium size	39	3
Societies with petty states or none	79	18

Null hypothesis: p = .066
Tendency A: strength 98%

single level of integration above that of the organized local community, as in the case of a paramount chief ruling over a small district embracing several villages.

Tests were also made of the association of spirit aggression theories with metal working and other examples of complex technological achievements, using comparative data from the *Ethnographic Atlas* (Murdock 1967). The coefficients were positive in all cases, but only in the case of loom-weaving did they attain the level of statistical significance (see Correlation 15).

Correlation 15

Spirit Aggression Theories with Loom-Weaving

	Spirit Aggression Theories Important	Spirit Aggression Theories Unimportant or Unreported
Weaving practiced on a true loom	58	5
Loom-weaving not practiced	56	13

Null hypothesis: p = .057
Tendency A: strength 96%

Correlation 16

Spirit Aggression Theories with Intensive Techniques of Cultivation

	Spirit Aggression Theories Important	Spirit Aggression Theories Absent or Unreported
Tillers employing intensive techniques of cultivation	37	2
Tillers not employing intensive techniques	51	11

Null hypothesis: p = .0005
Tendency A: strength 98%

Rather surprisingly, spirit aggression theories proved not to be associated significantly with the practice of agriculture. However, among agricultural societies, as reported in Column 28 of the *Ethnographic Atlas* (Murdock 1967), they were found to be positively correlated with the use of intensive techniques of cultivation, such as irrigation, crop rotation, and the application of fertilizers (see Correlation 16).

The foregoing correlations are perhaps not particularly illuminating since they seem to stem fairly directly from regional distributions. Paradoxes, however, will begin to emerge in Chapter X.

References Cited

Fortune, R. F. Omaha Secret Societies. Columbia University Contributions to Anthropology 15: 1–193. 1932.

Hart, D. M. The Aith Waryaghar of the Moroccan Rif. Tucson, 1976.

Murdock, G. P. Social Structure. New York, 1949.

———. Ethnographic Atlas. Pittsburgh, 1967.

Murdock, G. P., and C. Provost. Measurement of Cultural Complexity. Ethnology 12: 379–392. 1973.

X

Aggression and Its Projection

Until our research was well advanced, it was assumed that the principal supernatural theories of illness—those of witchcraft, sorcery, and spirit aggression—had a common denominator in the phenomenon of aggression. Overt human aggression was recognized from the outset as a leading natural cause of illness. Sorcery and witchcraft appeared to be obvious expressions of this basic impulse, and theories of spirit aggression seemed like direct products of its projection to the realm of the supernatural. If man creates spirits and gods in his own image—and he clearly does—he must necessarily endow them with similar impulses, and it requires no great stretch of the imagination to conceive of illness and other misfortunes as manifestations of the aggressive or punitive reactions of such beings.

It was apparent almost from the beginning that our inquiry into the factors determining theories of illness, particularly those involving supernatural causation, would be appreciably enhanced by new evidence bearing on the hypothesis of Whiting and Child (1953) that the projection of the personality consequences of child-training practices generates such explanations. A recent paper by Herbert Barry and associates, "Traits Inculcated in Childhood," (Barry et al. 1976) seemed especially promising in this respect because it provides coded data on the strength of the inculcation of a series of personality traits, including trust and aggressiveness, for all the societies of our own sample.

Unfortunately the usefulness of this paper is impaired by a series of technical errors: (1) the coding was distorted by an unconscious bias against using the top and bottom categories on a five-point scale, thereby reducing it in essence to a three-point scale; (2) in a reaction to this restriction the coders were encouraged to qualify the numerical codes by adding plus and minus signs, but without explicit guidelines, so that a second unconscious bias produced a distorted ratio of nearly thrice as many pluses as minuses; and (3) the original scale was arbitrarily expanded to a ten-point ordinal scale on the basis of unspecified but clearly invalid assumptions about the numerical value of the qualifying signs.

These distortions, fortunately, are readily corrected by omitting all plus and minus signs from the codes, thereby restoring the original scale on which the coders had made their judgments. Even with this adjustment, however, the ratings for the inculcation of trust could not be used to indicate a possible factor in the incidence of sorcery or witchcraft theories because the occurrence of these magical practices had been employed as a criterion for lowering the rating of trust.

Barry's ratings of the strength of the inculcation of aggressiveness seemed, on the other hand, to be ideally suited to a comparison with our own ratings of the importance of spirit aggression theories of illness. He devotes four columns in his table to rating the strength of the inculcation of aggressiveness—for boys in both early and late childhood and for girls during the same two periods. Omitting the plus and minus signs, we note that in 122 cases the strength of inculcation is rated lower than average, that is, with ratings of one or two, whereas in 45 instances it is rated higher than average (ratings of four or five). Comparison with our codes in Table 2 shows that 107 of the below-average cases but only 34 of the above-average cases are societies in which spirit aggression theories are predominant or of substantial subsidiary importance. In other words, weak early inculcation of aggressiveness is about three times as likely as strong inculcation to be correlated with (and hence presumably a cause of) projection of aggression to the supernatural level.

These data are obviously in irreconcilable conflict with the theoretical position of Whiting and Child (1953), from which one would anticipate a positive rather than a negative relationship between the strong inculcation and the projection of aggression. They also seem to flout common sense. On what imaginable grounds can one conceive that projected aggression should be strong precisely where inculcated aggressiveness is weak?

My initial impulse was to dismiss Barry's paper out of hand as leading to erroneous conclusions and to assign the blame to his failure to define aggressiveness and to his treatment of it as a "thing" with dimensions rather than as a reified construct. Reflection, however, stimulated by my respect for the experience and expertise of Barry's coders, led me to consider a more charitable possible interpretation. Perhaps, despite the defective methodology and inadequate supervision, the coders did uncover something significant. Conceivably the source of the seeming conflict lies in the incorrectness, not of the coded data nor of the Whiting-Child hypothesis concerning projection, but of my assumption that theories of what I have called "spirit aggression" are adequately accounted for as simple derivates (projections) from whatever it is in man's behavior that is commonly termed, however loosely, as "aggression."

My obvious next step was to intercorrelate the incidence of the three supernatural theories that had been assumed to be probable derivates of aggression, in order to determine the degree of their mutual dependence or independence. Correlation 6, which examines the relationship of witchcraft and sorcery theories, has already shown them to be negatively rather than positively correlated. In Correlations 17 and 18 both are similarly compared with spirit aggression theories.

The discovery from Correlation 6 that beliefs in the theories of witchcraft and sorcery are negatively rather than positively correlated, and indeed are essentially antithetical, is perhaps surprising, but the demonstration in Correlations 17 and 18 that both are negatively correlated with the incidence of theories of spirit aggression creates genuine astonishment. How could it possibly happen that three pre-

Correlation 17

Witchcraft Theories of Illness with Spirit Aggression Theories

	Witchcraft Theories Important	Witchcraft Theories Absent or Unimportant
Spirit aggression theories important	21	97
Spirit aggression theories unimportant or unreported	6	15

Null hypothesis: p = .194
Tendency B: strength 96%

Correlation 18

Sorcery Theories of Illness with Spirit Aggression Theories

	Sorcery Theories Important	Sorcery Theories Absent or Unimportant
Spirit aggression theories important	54	64
Spirit aggression theories unimportant or unreported	18	3

Null hypothesis: p = .00056
Tendency D: strength 98%

sumed derivatives from a common source could diverge so markedly from one another? If not actually impossible, such an occurrence is certainly statistically highly improbable. We are, therefore, driven to the conclusion that at least one and perhaps two of the three theories are profoundly influenced by projection from a source quite distinct from overt human aggression.

In the case of witchcraft theories it is difficult to sense any emotional concomitant other than unadulterated aggression in the form of malice, envy, or spite. In the case of sorcery theories, however, what a shaman's patients and his public observe of his magical activities are their beneficent rather than their maleficent results. We can, therefore, postulate, though we cannot prove, that the kinds of emotions which the recipient of magical therapy is likely to associate with his shaman should resemble those which any modern patient tends to associate with his physician, namely, qualified hope, apprehension, and gratitude.

The search for comparable emotional concomitants of spirit aggression theories will engage our attention in Chapter XI.

References Cited

Barry, H. III, L. Josephson, E. Lauer, and C. Marshall. Traits Inculcated in Childhood. Ethnology 15: 83–114. 1976.

Whiting, J. W. M., and I. L. Child. Child Training and Personality. New Haven, 1953.

XI

The Pastoral Relationship

In cross-cultural research, as in other applications of statistics to large numbers of cases, the hope is to discover trends in the data. One does not expect unanimity or perfect correlations and seldom encounters them. One such statistical gem did, however, come to light in the present study in the course of comparing the association of spirit aggression theories of illness with the major types of subsistence economy. Without exception, every society in the sample which depends primarily on animal husbandry for its economic livelihood regards spirit aggression as either the predominant or an important secondary cause of illness (see Correlation 19). The comparative data for this and all other correlations in this chapter are derived from the *Ethnographic Atlas* (Murdock 1967).

Correlation 19
Spirit Aggression Theories with Predominant Pastoralism

	Spirit Aggression Theories Important	Spirit Aggression Theories Unimportant or Unreported
Pastoralism the predominant type of food quest	12	0
Other types of food quest predominant	106	21

Null hypothesis: p = .128
Tendency A: strength 100%

Pastoral nomads are widely renowned for their warlike qualities and for careers of expansion and conquest. Notable cases include the Huns in Europe, the Mongols in Asia, the Bedouin Arabs in North Africa, the Fulani in West Africa, the Masai in East Africa, and the Apache in the American Southwest. Facts like these seemed to confirm my initial assumption that the theories of spirit aggression derive from an emphasis on aggression in daily life.

Further analysis, however, revealed a strong tendency for spirit aggression theories to occur in all societies that keep large domestic animals, agricultural as well as pastoral (see Correlation 20). Large

Correlation 20

Spirit Aggression Theories with Keeping of Large Domestic Animals

	Spirit Aggression Theories Important	Spirit Aggression Theories Unimportant or Unreported
Societies keeping large domestic animals	71	8
Societies lacking large domestic animals	47	13

Null hypothesis: p = .051
Tendency A: strength 94%

animals are to be understood here as including horses, cattle, water buffaloes, camels, reindeer, sheep, goats, and llamas, but not pigs, dogs, or household pets. The same tendency even appears in agricultural societies which harness their animals to the plow (see Correlation 21).

William Graham Sumner (1906: 6–7) has called attention to "the aleatory element in life, the element of risk and loss, good or bad fortune. This element is never absent from the affairs of men. It has greatly influenced their life philosophy and policy. On one side, good luck may mean something for nothing, the extreme case of prosperity

Correlation 21

Spirit Aggression Theories with Plow Cultivation

	Spirit Aggression Theories Important	Spirit Aggression Theories Unimportant or Unreported
Societies with plow cultivation	21	1
Agricultural societies lacking the plow	54	12

Null hypothesis: p = .107
Tendency A: strength 99%

and felicity. On the other side, ill luck may mean failure, loss, calamity, and disappointment, in spite of the most earnest and well-planned endeavor. . . . The aleatory element has always been the connecting link between the struggle for existence and religion. It is only by religious rites that the aleatory element in the struggle for existence could be controlled."

People whose capital consists largely of flocks and herds have vastly more at risk than those whose resources are invested in land. They can lose all they own almost overnight in an enemy attack, an unexpected drought, or an epidemic of rinderpest just as they can multiply their possessions by a successful raid. Their dependence on the protection and support of supernatural beings is, as they view the situation, extreme, and what they project to the supernatural level may well concern their sense of dependence even more than the aggressiveness with which they are prepared to defend their precious possessions.

Particularly impressive is the demonstration in Correlation 22 that societies which milk their domestic animals are especially likely to hold spirit aggression theories of illness. Only two societies, the Otoro (#30) and the Riffians (#42), are exceptions, and we already know from Carleton Coon that the low incidence of spirit aggression theories for the Riffians is a coding error.

Correlation 22

Spirit Aggression Theories with Milking of Domestic Animals

	Spirit Aggression Theories Important	Spirit Aggression Theories Unimportant or Unreported
Societies milking domestic animals	43	2
Societies not milking domestic animals	75	19

Null hypothesis: p = .0105
Tendency A: strength 99%

It may possibly contribute to our understanding to recognize that in milking we have an exact parallel to the foremost example of symbiosis in the field of ethology (the scientific study of animal behavior), namely, the propensity of certain species of insects for harboring in their nests insects of another species which exude a substance which their hosts consume with avidity. The parasites are kept, in short, for the "milk" which they produce.

It is not only that domestic animals provide transportation, power, meat, milk, wool, and other products in return for food, shelter, and protection. This reciprocity of services tends also to engender a measure of emotional mutuality, as I am aware from having spent my boyhood and youth on a subsistence farm where I interacted intimately not only with milch cows but also with draft oxen and riding, driving, and draft horses. My relations with all of them were characterized by a substantial measure of mutual confidence, respect, and even affection, coupled with a sense of *noblesse oblige*. Urbanized colleagues have scoffed at this as sentimental nonsense, but I am willing to refer the issue to any jury composed of ranchers, cowboys, and/or dairy farmers; of polo players, old cavalrymen, and/or grooms in racing stables; or of equestrian performers in horse shows, circuses, or rodeos.

This pastoral relationship of man with his domestic animals is certainly capable of generalization to the gods he worships, as is attested by what is surely the classic example of projection in all literature, a passage as symbolically meaningful to English speakers in the King James translation as it must have been to the ancient Hebrews themselves, namely, the Twenty-third Psalm: "The Lord is my shepherd; I shall not want. He maketh me to lie down in green pastures: he leadeth me beside the still waters. . . . Yea, though I walk through the valley of the shadow of death, I will fear no evil: for thou art with me; thy rod and thy staff they comfort me" (vs. 1-2, 4).

The question naturally arises whether the relationship between man and his domestic animals actually has a distinctive quality of its own or whether it is merely a special variant of the class of master-servant relationships prevailing among human beings. Is an animal basically a slave of man, or, expressed in reverse, is slavery essentially a form of animal husbandry in which human beings are the domestic animals? If so, slavery, which is reported in at least an incipient form for approximately half the societies of our sample, should reveal a similar association with spirit aggression theories of illness. The fact that Correlation 23 is negative, whereas all those involving animal husbandry are positive, argues strongly for the uniqueness of the pastoral relationship between man and his larger domestic animals.

Correlation 23
Spirit Aggression Theories with Slavery

	Spirit Aggression Theories Important	Spirit Aggression Theories Unimportant or Unreported
Slavery present in any form	50	12
Slavery totally absent	62	8

Null hypothesis: p = .153
Tendency D: strength 94%

In the literature the domestication of plants, particularly the cereal grains, is commonly treated as the crucial achievement of the Neolithic Revolution. To the extent, however, that the domestication of animals may have led ultimately to a new conception of the supernatural, it should probably be accorded at least equal historical importance.

References Cited

Murdock, G. P. Ethnographic Atlas. Pittsburgh, 1967.
Sumner, W. G. Folkways. Boston, 1906.

XII

Sin, Sex, and Sickness

The above title, borrowed from a paper by Hallowell (1939), aptly sets the scene for this chapter. Witchcraft, sorcery, and spirit aggression seemed, at least initially, to be concerned in varying ways with aggression. The theory of mystical retribution, on the other hand, appears to connote quite another emotional concept, that of guilt or a sense of sin, induced, as its definition implies, by "acts in violation of some taboo or moral injunction." As indicated in Table 3, theories of mystical retribution are reported for nearly 80 percent of the societies in our world sample and are rated as important (predominant or significant) in 28 percent of them. They thus rank as the third most widespread among the theories of supernatural causation.

For purposes of analysis a distinction should be drawn between taboos and other behavioral prohibitions. As Sumner (1906: 30) has intimated, taboos are negative mores, customary restrictions on modes of behavior that are deemed morally wrong. Along with positive standards of morality, they are normally internalized during the process of early socialization in the form of what is popularly termed the "conscience" of the individual members of a society. They are in a sense self-regulating, since they automatically exert an inner pressure toward conformity. The very thought of violation arouses a monitory "twinge" of conscience which is usually sufficient to suppress the prohibited behavior. If the impulse is strong enough to overcome this resistance and produce an actual breach of the taboo, the warning signal tends to be magnified into more acute "pangs" of guilt.

A behavioral restriction which lacks such internal support is ineffective unless bulwarked by penalties for violation imposed from without, but even then it is not self-regulating. From time immemorial political authorities have sought to control social behavior by official edicts or legislation, and invariably they have found it necessary to back them by special means of enforcement. Speed limits on modern superhighways, for example, are likely to be observed only when an enforcement officer is considered likely to be lurking around the next bend. A similar ineffectiveness characterized the Prohibition Amendment despite its incorporation in the highest law of the land.

The following passage on the Semang (#77) from an earlier work of mine (Murdock 1934: 103–04) demonstrates that even belief in the sponsorship of prohibitions by a supreme being is insufficient to assure their automatic observation when they seem arbitrary or devoid of ethical justification:

> Towering vastly above all the rest [of the gods] . . . looms Karei, the god of thunder. Invisible, superhuman in size, omnipotent, omniscient, he created men, gave them their souls, and is aware of their every transgression. Though sometimes kindly and well disposed, he grows angry when they do wrong and warns or slays them with his thunderbolts. Sin is the violation of a taboo imposed by Karei. The category of sins includes, curiously enough, not theft or murder, but such things as familiarity with one's mother-in-law, killing a sacred black wasp or certain tabooed birds, mocking a tame or helpless animal, sexual intercourse in the daytime, playing with birds' eggs, drawing water in a vessel blackened by fire, watching dogs mating, combing one's hair during a thunderstorm or the mourning period, and throwing a spear in the morning—quite permissible in the afternoon! The sound of thunder, the sign of Karei's anger, gives warning that someone has sinned. All who are conscious of guilt, or at least one person representing the band, must hasten to render atonement by a blood sacrifice.

It should be noted that the prevailing theory of illness among the Semang is coded in Table 2 as spirit aggression and not as mystical retribution. Only the latter has the self-regulating character of taboos.

There are at least two ways in which the violation of taboos can become conceptually linked with the causation of illness. One is through the psychological mechanism familiar to psychiatrists under the technical name of "conversion." Guilt can be extremely uncomfortable and even painful to the sufferer and hence is readily confused with or interpreted as a form of somatic illness. Many a surgeon has been induced to operate and many a physician to prescribe at the urging of patients whose imaginations have deceived them in this manner. It is by no means inconceivable that the same mechanism that produces conversion symptoms in neurotic or psychotic patients may also underlie mystical retribution theories of illness. Only the regional distribution of these theories renders this hypothesis suspect. Manifestations of guilt are exceptionally prominent in religious behavior in the Circum-Mediterranean region, as witness the Flagellants of medieval Europe and the evangelistic revivalism of modern Protestantism, but, as revealed in Table 3, the incidence of beliefs in mystical retribution is far lower in this region than anywhere else in the world.

An alternative explanation is suggested by the high morbidity and brief life expectancy of most of the indigenous peoples of the world. This assures that, by chance alone, the breach of a taboo will frequently be accompanied or shortly followed by some illness in the sinner. By *post hoc, ergo propter hoc* reasoning this is likely to be interpreted, especially if repeated, as a direct consequence of the violation.

In analyzing the other principal supernatural theories of illness, we were fortunate in having at our disposal substantial bodies of coded information on various aspects of technology, subsistence economy, and social organization which, when intercorrelated with the data in Table 2, give rise to insights of considerable interest and significance. They fail to yield comparable enlightenment, however, when examined in connection with the information on mystical retribution theories. The probable explanation is not hard to figure out: Economics, technology, and social organization are so distantly related to taboo violation and guilt that significant correlations are not really to be expected. What is needed is a corpus of coded data of a very different kind, for example, on the definition and punishment of various torts and crimes, on moral codes and their sanctions, on recognized grounds for divorce or separation, and on such behavioral manifestations of sin as confession and expiation. Unfortunately, to my knowledge coded information on these subjects simply does not exist.

On the other hand, a modest amount of coded information is available on a related subject, the regulation of sex, which is well known to be intimately associated with anxiety and guilt. Especially pertinent is a code on "Norms of Premarital Sex Behavior," Column 78 in the *Ethnographic Atlas* (Murdock 1967). Its categories are dichotomized in Correlation 24 for comparison with the data in Table 2 on the incidence and significance of theories of mystical retribution. It should be noted of this correlation, first, that it is positive in sign rather than negative as might have been expected and, second, that it does not attain the level of statistical significance.

Correlation 24
Mystical Retribution Theories with Premarital Sex Freedom

	Mystical Retribution Theories Important	Mystical Retribution Theories Absent or Unimportant
Premarital sex relations common and subject only to weak sanctions or none	24	55
Premarital sex relations prohibited, strongly sanctioned, and rare in fact	5	19

Null hypothesis: p = .26
Tendency B: strength 95%

A second body of coded data, presented in Barry et al. (1976), records the relative strength of the inculcation, during childhood, of sexual restraints on masturbation, heterosexual play, and comparable erotic behavior. The comparison of these data with the incidence of mystical retribution theories yields results consistent with those in Correlation 24, namely, a positive but nonsignificant correlation with weak inculcation rather than, as anticipated, with strong inculcation.

The evidence at our disposal is unfortunately too scanty and equivocal to contribute substantially to the understanding of mystical retribution theories of the causation of illness. It does, however, tell us something about the range and distribution of patterns of human sexuality. From Column 78 of the *Ethnographic Atlas* we learn that norms of premarital sex behavior vary between extremes of strictness and laxity defined as follows: (A) "Premarital sex relations prohibited, strongly sanctioned, and in fact rare." Reported for twenty-six societies in our world sample. (Z) "Premarital sex relations freely permitted and subject to no sanctions." Reported for sixteen societies. The remaining societies of the sample fall into intermediate categories which lean more toward the lax than to the strict extreme. A slight majority of the societies in the Circum-Mediterranean region are coded at the strict extreme, which most readers will recognize as according with the traditional Judeo-Christian standard of sexual ethics. Equally familiar, and widely publicized, are the trends toward relaxation that have developed in Western society during the course of the present century and are widely though dubiously attributed to the influence of Sigmund Freud. These are manifested in the increasing rates of divorce, cohabitation without marriage, and illegitimacy and in the vocal advocacy of gay rights, women's lib, and liberalized abortion.

Far less is generally known about the circumstances and concomitants of complete freedom at the lax end of the sexual spectrum. Do these societies actually realize the hope and expectation of liberals that anxiety and guilt over sex should be substantially reduced by sexual freedom and that a man's mental health and level of happiness should be correspondingly enhanced? Evidence bearing on precisely this point is available for one of the societies of our sample, the Trukese (#109) of the central Pacific.

In 1947 I led a party of younger colleagues on an ethnographic field investigation in Truk. To acquire a facility in the native language, each member of the party attached himself to a young man in his late teens or early twenties who became his linguistic informant and constant companion. These lads also assisted in housekeeping chores, notably in the collective preparation of the daily evening meal, an occasion marked by lighthearted conversation, joking, and anecdotes revolving largely around the subject of sex. From observations in this and other contexts, it became apparent that Trukese youth are no less preoccupied with sex—and frustrated in its pursuit—than are adolescents in our own society. And this despite the fact that sexual intercourse carries no moral stigma and is universally engaged in by boys from about the age of sixteen and by girls from the onset of puberty. This seeming paradox has been explored by Goodenough (1949), whose interest was first aroused as a result of his assignment as the field party's master chef.

Experimentation with sex is not attended by guilt feelings in Truk. It is involved, however, with a strong sense of modesty about genital exposure, which requires strict privacy during the performance of the sex act. This is difficult to achieve out-of-doors and in the daytime because of the relative density of the population and the sparsity of vegetation cover, so that intercourse, when it occurs, is usually furtive, hasty, and less-than-fully satisfying. At night it normally takes place in the dwelling of the girl's extended family because of the danger of lurking supernaturals outdoors, and it must be performed so quietly as not to awaken the other inmates. In particular, it should not disturb the girl's father, for this would be most embarrassing in view of the taboo relationship prevailing in Truk between father and daughter. A further complicating fact is that females are prone to be critical of male performance and to ridicule any failure in timing or technique.

Goodenough (1949: 620) concludes his extended analysis as follows:

The situation on Truk demonstrates that permissive attitudes and a relatively frank approach to sexual intercourse do not necessarily result in lowered preoccupation with sex or preclude an idealization of romantic love. If sociological and other situational factors frustrate the achievement of those goals which the permissiveness of the culture leads one to anticipate, preoccupation with them is likely to result. It is also clear that the many aspects of a people's behavior cannot be explained as functions of some one variable, such as permissiveness, which appears as only one of several conditioning factors.

In view of the complexity of the attendant circumstances, we should perhaps not have expected the coded data on premarital sexuality to have revealed unambiguous correlations with theories of the causation of illness. However, in partial recompense, they do enable us to test what is perhaps the first behavioral science theory propounded in the history of man. Herodotus (ca. 484–425 B.C.), who is variously claimed as the "father" of history, of geography, and of anthropology, hypothesized that peoples who live in warmer climates tend to be sexually more active and less restrained than those who inhabit the temperate and frigid zones. This theory has been cited and discussed, usually with considerable skepticism, by hundreds of subsequent philosophers and social scientists, but none has hitherto been able to check its accuracy against the cultural facts. This is done herewith in Correlation 25 by relating the previously cited data on norms of premarital sex behavior to the geographical coordinates listed in the appendix and adding comparable information obtained on 21 other societies in the original world sample of 188. Societies located between twenty-three degrees north and south latitude are compared with those residing outside the tropical zone. It is both gratifying and amusing to learn that, however sound or dubious his reasoning may have been, Herodotus has finally, after the lapse of some twenty-four hundred years, had his hypothesis confirmed.

Correlation 25
Sexuality and Climatic Zones

	Lax Premarital Sex Norms	Strict Premarital Sex Norms
Residents of the tropical zone	62	13
Residents of the temperate and frigid zones	32	19

Null hypothesis: p = .011
Tendency A: strength 90%

References Cited

Barry, H., L. Josephson, E. Lauer, and C. Marshall. Traits Inculcated in Childhood. Ethnology 15: 83–114. 1976.

Goodenough, W. H. Premarital Freedom on Truk: Theory and Practice. American Anthropologist 51: 615–620. 1949.

Hallowell, A. I. Sin, Sex and Sicknesss in Saulteaux Belief. British Journal of Medical Psychology 18: 191–197. 1939.

Murdock, G. P. Our Primitive Contemporaries. New York, 1934.

———. Ethnographic Atlas. Pittsburgh, 1967.

Sumner, W. G. Folkways. Boston, 1906.

APPENDIX

INDEX

APPENDIX

The Societies Surveyed:
Identification and Bibliography

The 139 societies from which ethnographic data have been drawn for this study are listed below in numerical order. Most of them are from the standard sample of the world's cultures adopted by the Cross-Cultural Coding Center at the University of Pittsburgh. An "a" following a number indicates that the society is an alternative to one in the standard sample. Identifying information is supplied for each society under the following symbols:

P   The pinpointed subgroup to which the data primarily pertain
G   The geographical coordinates for the center of the society's territory
T   The approximate date to which the data specifically relate

The principal ethnographic sources for each society are listed in alphabetical order of authors following the identification. For readers primarily interested in theories of illness an asterisk (*) is placed before the sources that contain the fullest information on the subject. For those more interested in the cultural context a number of sources have been included which contain little information on illness but substantial data on other aspects of culture. These are marked by a dagger (†).

1. Nama Hottentot. P: Gei //Khauan tribe. G: 27°30'S, 17°E. T: 1860.
    *Hoernlé, A. W. Certain Rites of Transition and the Conception of !nau among the Hottentots. Harvard African Studies 2: 65–82. 1918.
    *Schapera, I. The Khoisan Peoples of South Africa. London, 1930.
    †Schultze, L. Aus Namaland und Kalahari. Jena, 1907.
2. Kung Bushmen. P: Nyae Nyae region. G: 19°50'S, 20°35'E. T: 1950.
    †Marshall, L. Marriage among the !Kung Bushmen. Africa 29: 335–364. 1954.
    *———. !Kung Bushman Religious Beliefs. Africa 32: 221–252. 1962.

*————. The !Kung Bushmen of the Kalahari Desert. Peoples of Africa, ed. J. L. Gibbs, Jr., pp. 241–278. New York, 1965.

Schapera, I. The Khoisan Peoples of South Africa. London, 1930.

3. Thonga. P: Ronga subtribe. G: 25°50'S, 32°20'E. T: 1895.

*Junod, H. A. The Life of a South African Tribe. 2d ed. 2 vols. London, 1927.

5. Mbundu. P: Bailundo subtribe. G: 12°15'S, 16°30'E. T: 1890.

*Childs, G. M. Umbundu Kinship and Character. London, 1949.

†Edwards, A. C. The Ovimbundu under Two Sovereignties. London, 1962.

*Hambly, W. D. The Ovimbundu of Angola. Field Museum Anthropology Series 21: 89–362. 1934.

McCulloch, M. The Ovimbundu of Angola. London, 1952.

6. Suku. P: "lineage center" in Feshi territory. G: 6°S, 18°E. T: 1920.

†Holemans, K. Etudes sur alimentation en milieu coutumier du Kwango. Annales de la Société Belge de Médecine Tropicale 39: 361–374. 1959.

Kopytoff, I. Family and Lineage among the Suku. The Family Estate in Africa, ed. R. F. Gray and P. H. Gulliver, pp. 83–116. Boston, 1964.

*————. The Suku of Southwestern Congo. Peoples of Africa, ed. J. L. Gibbs, Jr., pp. 441–477. New York, 1965.

8. Nyakyusa. P: age village near Mwaya and Masoko. G: 9°30'S, 34°E. T: 1934.

*Wilson, G. An Introduction to Nyakyusa Society. Bantu Studies 10: 253–292. 1936.

*Wilson, M. Good Company. London, 1951.

†————. Rituals of Kinship among the Nyakyusa. London, 1957.

9. Hadza. G: 3°45'S, 35°E. T: 1930.

†Bleek, D. F. The Hadzapi or Watindiga. Africa 4: 273–285. 1911.

*Kohl-Larsen, L. Wildbeuter in Ostafrika. Berlin, 1958.

*Woodburn, J. The Social Organization of the Hadza. Ph.D. dissertation, University of Cambridge, 1964.

11a. Chagga. G: 3°30'S, 38°E. T: 1906.

Dundas, C. Kilima-Njaro and Its Peoples. London, 1924.

*Gutmann, B. Das Recht der Dschagga. Arbeiten zur Entwicklungspsychologie 7: 1–778. 1926.

*Raum, O. F. Chaga Childhood. London, 1940.

12. Ganda. P: Kyaddondo district. G: 0°20'N, 32°30'E. T: 1875.

Kagwa, A. The Customs of the Baganda. New York, 1934.

†Mair, L. An African People in the Twentieth Century. London, 1934.

Murdock, G. P. Our Primitive Contemporaries, pp. 508–550. New York, 1934.

*Roscoe, J. The Baganda. London, 1911.

13. Mbuti Pygmies. P: net hunters of the Epulu group. G: 1°45′N, 28°20′E. T: 1950.

Putnam, P. The Pygmies of the Ituri Forest. A Reader in General Anthropology, ed. C. S. Coon, pp. 322–342. New York, 1938.

Turnbull, C. N. The Forest People. New York, 1961.

*————. Wayward Servants. New York, 1965.

*————. The Mbuti Pygmies. Anthropological Papers, American Museum of Natural History 50: iii, 1–282. 1965.

14. Nkundo Mongo. P: Ilanga group. G: 0°45′S, 19°E. T: 1930.

†Brepoels, H. Het familiehoofd bij de Nkundo negers. Congo 11: ii, 332–340. 1930.

*Hulstaert, G. Le mariage des Nkundó. Mémoires de l'Institut Royal Colonial Belge 8: 1–520. 1938.

15. Banen. P: Ndiki subtribe. G: 4°40′N, 19°E. T: 1935.

*Dugast, I. Monographie de la tribu des Ndiki. Travaux et Mémoires de l'Institut d'Ethnologie 58: ii, 1–635. 1959.

McCulloch, M., M. Littlewood, and I. Dugast. Peoples of the Central Cameroons. London, 1954.

16. Tiv. P: tar of Benue province. G: 7°15′N, 9°E. T: 1920.

Abraham, R. C. The Tiv People. Lagos, 1933.

*Bohannan, P., and L. Bohannan. The Tiv of Central Nigeria. London, 1953.

*————. Three Source Books in Tiv Ethnography. New Haven, 1958.

Downes, R. M. The Tiv Tribe. Kaduna, 1933.

*East, R., ed. Akiga's Story. London, 1939.

18: Fon. P: city and environs of Abomey. G: 7°12′N, 1°56′E. T: 1890.

Argyle, W. J. The Fon of Dahomey. London, 1966.

*Herskovits, M. J. Dahomey. 2 vols. New York, 1938.

*Herskovits, M. J., and F. S. Herskovits. An Outline of Dahomean Religious Belief. Memoirs, American Anthropological Association 41: 1–77. 1933.

Le Herissé, A. L'ancien royaume du Dahomey. Paris, 1911.

19. Ashanti. P: Kumasi state. G: 7°N, 1°30′W. T: 1895.

Fortes, M. Kinship and Marriage among the Ashanti. African Systems of Kinship and Marriage, ed. A. R. Radcliffe-Brown and D. Forde, pp. 252–284. London, 1950.

*Lystad, R. A. The Ashanti. New Brunswick, 1958.

Rattray, R. S. Ashanti. Oxford, 1923.

*————. Religion and Art in Ashanti. Oxford, 1927.

20. Mende. P: vicinity of the town of Bo. G: 7°50′N, 12°W. T: 1945.

*Little, K. L. The Mende of Sierra Leone. London, 1951.

McCulloch, M. The Peoples of Sierra Leone Protectorate. London, 1950.

†Staub, J. Beiträge zur Kenntnis der materiellen Kultur der Mendi. Solothurn, 1936.

21. Wolof. P: Upper and Lower Salum in the Gambia. G: 13°45′N, 12°W. T: 1950.

*Ames, D. W. Plural Marriage among the Wolof. Ph.D. dissertation, Northwestern University, 1953.

*Gamble, D. P. The Wolof of Senegambia. London, 1957.

23. Tallensi. G: 10°40′N, 0°35′W. T: 1934.

*Fortes, M. The Dynamics of Clanship among the Tallensi. London, 1945.

*——. The Web of Kinship among the Tallensi. London, 1949.

†Fortes, M., and S. L. Fortes. Food in the Domestic Economy of the Tallensi. Africa 9: 237–276. 1936.

Rattray, R. S. Tribes of the Ashanti Hinterland. Oxford, 1932.

24. Songhai. P: Bamba division. G: 16°40′N, 2°40′W. T: 1940.

*Miner, H. The Primitive City of Timbuctoo. Princeton, 1953.

*Rouch, J. Les Songhay. Paris, 1954.

25. Fulani. P: Wodaabe of Niger. G: 15°N, 7°E. T: 1951.

*Dupire, M. Peuls nomades. Travaux et Mémoires de l'Institut d'Ethnologie 64: 1–327. 1962.

*——. The Position of Women in a Pastoral Society. Women of Tropical Africa, ed. D. Paulme, pp. 47–92. London, 1963.

Hopen, C. E. The Pastoral Fulani Family in Gwandu. London, 1958.

Stenning, D. J. Savannah Nomads. London, 1959.

26. Hausa. P: Zazzagawa. G: 10°30′N, 7°30′E. T: 1900.

*Greenberg, J. H. The Influence of Islam on a Sudanese Religion. Monographs of the American Ethnological Society 10: 1–73. 1946.

*——. Islam and Clan Organization among the Hausa. Southwestern Journal of Anthropology 3: 193–211. 1947.

*Smith, M. F. Baba of Karo. New York, 1955.

†Smith, M. G. The Economy of Hausa Communities of Zaria. Colonial Office Research Studies 16: 1–264. 1955.

27. Massa. P: in Cameroon. G: 10°20′N, 15°30′E. T: 1910.

Garine, I. de. Les Massa du Cameroun. Paris, 1964.

*Hagen, G. von. Die Bana. Baessler-Archiv 2: 77–116. 1912.

*Lembezat, B. Les populations païennes du Nord-Cameroun. Paris, 1961.

28. Azande. P: Yambio chiefdom. G: 5°N, 28°15′E. T: 1905.

Baxter, P. T. W., and A. Butt. The Azande and Related Peoples. London, 1953.

*Evans-Pritchard, E. E. Witchcraft, Oracles and Magic among the Azande. Oxford, 1937.

Larkin, G. M. An Account of the Azande. Sudan Notes and Records 9: 235–247; 10: 85–134. 1926–27.

Seligman, C. G., and B. Z. Seligman. Pagan Tribes of the Nilotic Sudan. London, 1932.

30. Otoro. G: 11°20'N, 30°40'E. T: 1930.

*Nadel, S. F. The Nuba. London, 1947.

31. Shilluk. G: 9°45'N, 31°30'E. T: 1910.

*Hofmayr, W. Die Schilluk. Vienna, 1925.

*Seligman, C. G., and B. Z. Seligman. Pagan Tribes of the Nilotic Sudan. London, 1932.

Westermann, D. The Shilluk People. Berlin, 1912.

32. Mao. P: northern division. G: 9°20'N, 34°40'E. T: 1939.

*Grottanelli, V. I. I Mao. Missione etnografica nel Uollaga Occidentale 1: 1–387. Rome, 1940.

33. Kaffa. G: 7°15'N, 36°15'E. T: 1905.

*Bieber, F. J. Kaffa. 2 vols. Münster, 1920–23.

†Huntingford, G. W. B. The Kingdoms of Kafa and Janjero. London, 1955.

34a. Dorobo. P: North Tindiret Forest band. G: 0°10'N, 35°30'E. T: 1927.

Huntingford, G. W. B. The Social Organization of the Dorobo. African Studies 1: 183–200. 1942.

———. The Social Institutions of the Dorobo. Anthropos 46: 1–48. 1951.

*———. The Political Organization of the Dorobo. Anthropos 49: 123–148. 1954.

36. Somali. P: Dolbahanta subtribe. G: 9°N, 47°E. T: 1900.

Lewis, I. M. Peoples of the Horn of Africa. London, 1955.

*———. A Pastoral Democracy. London, 1961.

Puccioni, N. Antropologia e etnographia delle genti della Somalia. Bologna, 1936.

37. Amhara. P: Gondar district. G: 13°30'N, 37°E. T: 1953.

*Messing, S. D. The Highland-Plateau Amhara of Ethiopia. Ph.D. dissertation, University of Pennsylvania, 1957.

39. Kenuzi Nubians. P: Kenuzi of Dahmit. G: 23°N, 38°45'E. T: 1900.

*Callender, C., and F. El Guindi. Life-Crisis Rituals among the Kenuz. Cleveland, 1971.

Herzog, R. Die Nubier. Berlin, 1957.

*Kennedy, J. G. Struggle for Change in a Nubian Community. Palo Alto, 1977.

40. Teda. P: Nomads of Tibesti. G: 21°30′N, 17°30′E. T: 1950.

   *Chapelle, J. Nomades noirs du Sahara. Paris, 1957.

   Cline, W. The Teda of Tibesti, Borku and Kawar. General Series in Anthropology 12: 1–52. 1950.

41. Tuareg. P: Ahaggaren. G: 23°N, 6°30′E. T: 1900.

   Benhazera, M. Six mois chez les Touareg de Ahaggar. Alger, 1908.

   *Lhote, H. Les Touaregs du Hoggar. Paris, 1955.

   *Nicolaisen, J. Ecology and Culture of the Pastoral Tuareg. Natioalmuseets Skrifter, Etnografisk Raeke 9: 1–540. Copenhagen, 1963.

42. Riffians. G: 35°N, 3°15′W. T: 1926.

   *Coon, C. S. Tribes of the Rif. Harvard African Studies 9: 1–417. 1931.

   Hart, D. M. The Aith Waryaghar of the Moroccan Rif. Tucson, 1976.

43. Egyptians. P: town and environs of Silwa. G: 24°45′N, 33°E. T: 1950.

   *Ammar, H. Growing Up in an Egyptian Village. London, 1954.

   Blackman, W. S. The Fellahin of Upper Egypt. London, 1927.

44. Hebrews. P: kingdom of Judah. G: 31°10′N, 35°E. T: 621 B.C.

   *Bright, J. A History of Israel. Philadelphia, 1959.

   *Dalman, G. Arbeit und Sitte in Palestina. 8 vols. Gütersloh, 1932.

   DeVaux, R. Ancient Israel. New York, 1961.

   †Forbes, R. J. Studies in Ancient Technology. 2d rev. ed. 9 vols. Leiden, 1964.

   *Noth, M. The Ancient Testament World. 4th ed. Philadelphia, 1966.

45. Babylonians. P: city and environs of Babylon. G: 32°35′N, 44°45′E. T: 1750 B.C.

   Delaporte, L. J. Mesopotamia. New York, 1925.

   †Driver, G. R., and J. C. Miles. The Babylonian Laws. 2 vols. Oxford, 1952–1955.

   Gadd, C. J. Hammurabi and the End of His Dynasty. Cambridge Ancient History, rev. ed., fascicle 35. Cambridge, 1965.

   *Saggs, H. W. F. The Greatness That Was Babylon. London, 1962.

   *———. Everyday Life in Babylonia and Assyria. New York, 1965.

46. Rwala Bedouin. G: 31°45′N, 28°30′E. T: 1913.

   *Musil, A. The Manners and Customs of the Rwala Bedouins. New York, 1928.

   Raswan, C. R. Black Tents of Arabia. New York, 1944.

47. Turks. P: Anatolian plateau. G: 39°20′N, 34°E. T: 1950.

   *Makal, M. A Village in Anatolia. London, 1954.

   *Pierce, J. E. Life in a Turkish Village. London, 1964.

*Stirling, P. Turkish Village. London, 1964.

48. Albanians. P: Gheg. G: 42°N, 20°E. T: 1910.

   *Coon, C. S. The Mountain of Giants. Papers, Peabody Museum of Archaeology and Ethnology, Harvard University 23: iii, 1–105. 1950.

   *Durham, M. E. High Albania. London, 1909.

   *———. Some Tribal Origins, Laws and Customs of the Balkans. London, 1928.

   Hasluck, M. The Unwritten Law in Albania. Cambridge, 1954.

49. Romans. P: city and environs of Rome. G: 41°50'N, 13°30'E. T: A.D. 110.

   *Balsdon, J. P. V. D. Life and Leisure in Ancient Rome. New York, 1969.

   Carcopino, J. Daily Life in Ancient Rome, ed. H. T. Howell. New Haven, 1940.

   *Friedländer, L. Roman Life and Manners under the Early Empire. London, 1908.

   Glover, T. R. Conflict of Religions in the Early Roman Empire. London, 1927.

   *Grant, M. The World of Rome. London, 1960.

   †Maxey, M. Occupations of the Lower Classes in Roman Society. Chicago, 1938.

   *Paoli, V. E. Rome: Its Peoples, Life and Customs. New York, 1963.

50. Basques. P: village of Vera de Bidasoa in Spain. G: 43°15'N, 1°40'W. T: 1940.

   *Caro Baroja, J. La vida rural en Vera de Bidasoa. Madrid, 1944.

   *———. Los Vascos. Madrid, 1958.

   Douglass, W. A. Death in Murelaga. Seattle, 1969.

51a. Scots. P: Isle of Lewis. G: 58°15'N, 6°40'W. T: 1950.

   Ducey, P. R. Cultural Continuity and Population Change in the Isle of Skye. Ph.D. dissertation. Columbia University, 1956.

   *Geddes, A. The Isle of Lewis and Harris. Edinburgh, 1955.

   Parman, S. M. Sociocultural Change in a Scottish Crofting Township. Ph.D. dissertation, Rice University, 1972.

   *Thompson, F. G. Harris and Lewis: Outer Hebrides. Rev. ed. London, 1973.

52. Lapps. P: Könkämä district. G: 68°40'N, 21°30'E. T: 1950.

   *Bernatzig, H. A. Overland with the Nomad Lapps. New York, 1955.

   *Karsten, R. The Religion of the Samek. Leiden, 1955.

   Pehrson, R. N. The Bilateral Network of Social Relations in Könkämä Lapp District. Indiana University Publications, Slavic and East European Series 5: 1–128. 1957.

   *Turi, J. Turi's Book of Lapland. New York, 1931.

*Whitaker, I. Social Relations in a Nomadic Lappish Community. Uitgitt af Norsk Folkmuseum 2: 1–114. 1955.

53. Samoyed. P: Yurak. G: 68°N, 52°E. T: 1894.

*Donner, K. Among the Samoyed in Siberia. New Haven, 1954.

Englehardt, E. A. A Russian Province of the North. Westminster, 1899.

Hajdu, P. Samoyed Peoples and Languages. Indiana University Publications, Uralic and Altaic Series 14: 1–114. 1963.

Islavin, V. Samoiedy v domashnem i obschchestvennom bytu. St. Petersburg, 1947.

Jackson, F. G. The Great Frozen Land. London, 1895.

*Kopytoff, I. The Samoyed. New Haven, 1955.

57. Kurd. P: town and vicinity of Rowanduz. G: 36°30′N, 44°30′E. T: 1951.

Hansen, H. H. The Kurdish Woman's Life. Copenhagen Ethnographic Museum Record 7: 1–213. 1961.

†Leach, E. R. Social and Economic Organization of the Rowanduz Kurds. London School of Economics Monographs on Social Anthropology 3: 1–74. 1938.

*Masters, W. M. Rowanduz. Ph.D. dissertation, University of Michigan, 1953.

60. Gond. P: Hill Maria. G: 19°40′N, 80°50′E. T: 1930.

*Grigson, W. V. The Maria Gonds of Bastar. London, 1938.

61. Toda. G: 11°30′N, 76°30′E. T: 1900.

†Marshall, W. E. A Phrenologist amongst the Todas. London, 1873.

Murdock, G. P. Our Primitive Contemporaries, pp. 107–154. New York, 1934.

*Rivers, W. H. R. The Todas. London, 1906.

63. Uttar Pradesh. P: village and vicinity of Senapur. G: 25°55′N, 83°E. T: 1945.

*Dube, S. C. Cultural Factors in Rural Community Development. Journal of Asian Studies 16: 19–30. 1956.

*Luschinsky, M. S. The Life of Women in a Village of North India. Ph.D. dissertation, Cornell University, 1963.

65. Kazak. P: Great Horde. G: 42°N, 65°E. T: 1885.

*Castagné, J. Magie et exorcisme chez les Kazak-Kirghizes. Revue des Etudes Islamiques 4: 53–156. 1930.

*Grodekov, N. I. Kirghizy i Karakirghizy sur Dar'inskoi oblasti. Tashkent, 1889.

†Hudson, A. E. Kazak Social Structure. Yale University Publications in Anthropology 20: 1–109. 1938.

Radloff, W. Aus Sibirien. 2 vols. Leipzig, 1893.

66. Khalka Mongols. P: Narobanchin territory. G: 47°10′N, 96°E. T: 1920.

Ballis, W. B., ed. Mongolian People's Republic. 3 vols. New Haven, 1956.

*Maiskii, I. Sovremennaia Mongolia. Ordelenie, 1921.

Vreeland, H. H. Mongol Community and Kinship Structure. New Haven, 1954.

68. Lepcha. P: Lingthem and vicinity. G: 27°30′N, 89°E. T: 1937.

Das, A. K., and S. K. Banerjee. The Lepchas of Darjeeling District. Calcutta, 1962.

*Gorer, G. Himalayan Village. London, 1938.

Morris, J. Living with Lepchas. London, 1938.

69. Garo. P: village and environs of Rengsanggri. G: 26°N, 91°E. T: 1955.

*Burling, R. Rengsanggri. Philadelphia, 1963.

Playfair, A. The Garos. London, 1909.

71. Burmese. P: village of Nondwin. G: 22°N, 95°40′E. T: 1960.

Brohm, J. Buddhism and Animism in a Burmese Village. Journal of Asian Studies 22: 155–167. 1963.

*Nash, M. The Golden Road to Modernity. New York, 1965.

*Scott, J. G. The Burman: His Life and Notions. London, 1882.

†Trager,F. N., ed. Burma. 3 vols. New Haven, 1956.

72. Lamet. P: northwestern Laos. G: 20°N, 100°40′E. T: 1940.

*Izikowitz, K. G. Lamet. Ethnologiska Studier 17: 1–375. Göteborg, 1951.

73. Vietnamese. N: Red River delta in Tonkin. G: 20°30′N, 106°15′E. T: 1930.

Cadiére, L. M., et al. Vietnamese Ethnographic Papers. New Haven, 1953.

†Gourou, P. Les paysans du delta tonkinois. Paris, 1936.

*Hickey, G. C. Village in Vietnam. New Haven, 1964.

Langrand, G. Vie sociale et religieuse en Annam. Lille, 1945.

74. Rhade. P: village of Ko-sier. G: 13°N, 108°E. T: 1962.

*Donoghue, J. D., D. D. Whitney, and I. Ishino. People in the Middle. East Lansing, 1962.

*Sabatier, L. Recueil des coutumes rhadées du Darlac. Hanoi, 1940.

76. Siamese. P: village of Bang Chan. G: 14°N, 100°50′E. T: 1955.

Anuman Rajadhon, P. Life and Ritual in Old Siam, ed. W. J. Gedney. New Haven, 1961.

†Benedict, R. F. Thai Culture and Behavior. Ithaca, 1946.

*Hanks, J. R. Maternity and Its Rituals in Bang Chan. Ithaca, 1963.

Phillips, H. P. Thai Peasant Personality. Berkeley, 1965.

Sharp, R. L., H. M. Hauck, K. Janlekha, and R. B. Textor. Siamese Village. Bangkok, 1954.

77. Semang. P: Jahai subtribe. G: 5°N, 101°15′. T: 1925.

Evans, I. H. N. The Negritos of Malaya. Cambridge, 1937.

Murdock, G. P. Our Primitive Contemporaries, pp. 85–106. New York, 1934.

*Schebesta, P. Among the Forest Dwarfs of Malaya. London, 1927.

*———. Die Negrito Asiens. Studia Instituti Anthropos, vols. 6, 12, 13. Vienna, 1952–57.

78. Nicobarese. P: northern islands. G: 8°45′N, 92°50′E. T: 1870.

*Man, E. H. The Nicobar Islanders. Journal of the Royal Anthropological Institute 18: 354–394. 1888.

†Svoboda, W. Die Bewohner des Nikobaren-Archipels. Internationales Archiv für Ethnographie 5: 149–168. 1892–93.

*Whitehead, G. In the Nicobar Islands. London, 1924.

79. Andamanese. P: Aka-Bea tribe. G: 11°50′N, 93°E. T: 1860.

*Man, E. H. On the Aboriginal Inhabitants of the Andaman Islands. London, 1932.

*Radcliffe-Brown, A. R. The Andaman Islanders. Cambridge, 1922.

81. Tanala. P: Menabe subtribe. G: 20°S, 48°E. T: 1925.

*Linton, R. The Tanala. Field Museum of Natural History Anthropological Series 22: 1–334. 1933.

83. Javanese. P: vicinity of Pare. G: 7°43′S, 112°13′E. T: 1955.

*Geertz, C. The Religion of Java. Chicago, 1960.

*Geertz, H. The Javanese Family. New York, 1961.

Jay, R. R. Religion and Politics in Central Java. New Haven, 1963.

———. Javanese Villagers. Cambridge, 1969.

Koentjaraningrat. The Javanese of South Central Java. Social Structure in Southeast Asia, ed. G. P. Murdock, pp. 88–115. Chicago, 1960.

84. Balinese. P: village of Tihingan. G: 8°30′S, 115°20′E. T: 1958.

Belo, J. Traditional Balinese Culture. New York, 1970.

*Covarrubias, M. The Island of Bali. New York, 1937.

Franken, H. J., R. Goris, C. J. Grader, V. E. Korn, and J. L. Swellengrebel. Bali: Studies in Life, Thought and Ritual. The Hague, 1960.

Geertz, C. Tihingan. Villages in Indonesia, ed. Koentjaraningrat, pp. 210–293. Ithaca, 1967.

85. Iban. P: Ulu Ai group. G: 2°N, 113°E. T: 1950.

Freeman, J. S. Report on the Iban of Sarawak. Kuching, 1955.

†———. The Family System of the Iban. Cambridge Papers in Social Anthropology 1: 15–52. 1958.

*Gomes, E. H. Seventeen Years among the Sea Dyaks of Borneo. London, 1911.

*Howell, W. The Sea Dyak. Sarawak Gazette, vols. 38–50. 1908–10.

86. Badjau. P: Tawi-Tawi and adjacent islands. G: 5°N, 120°E. T: 1963.

Nimmo, H. A. Social Organization of the Tawi-Tawi Badjaw. Ethnology 4: 421–439. 1965.

*————. The Structure of Badjau Society. Ph.D. dissertation, University of Hawaii, 1969.

————. Badjau Sex and Reproduction. Ethnology 9: 251–262. 1970.

87. Toradja. P: Bare'e subgroup. G: 2°S, 121°E. T: 1910.

*Adriani, N., and A. C. Kruijt. De Bare'e-sprekende Toradja's. 3 vols. Batavia, 1912.

*Downs, R. E. The Religion of the Bare'e-speaking Toradja. The Hague, 1956.

89. Alorese. P: Atimelang. G: 8°20'S, 124°40'E. T: 1938.

DuBois, C. Attitude toward Food and Hunger in Alor. Language, Culture and Personality, ed. L. Spier et al., pp. 272–281. Menasha, 1941.

*————. The People of Alor. Minneapolis, 1944.

————. The Alorese. Psychological Frontiers of Society, ed. A. Kardiner, pp. 101–145. New York, 1945.

90. Tiwi. P: Melville Island. G: 11°20'S, 131°E. T: 1929.

†Goodale, J. C. Marriage Contracts among the Tiwi. Ethnology 1: 452–466. 1962.

*————. Tiwi Wives. Seattle, 1971.

Hart, A. C. M., and A. R. Pilling. The Tiwi of North Australia. New York, 1960.

*Mountford, C. P. The Tiwi, Their Arts and Ceremony. London, 1958.

*Pilling, A. R. Law and Feud in an Aboriginal Society of North Australia. Ph.D. dissertation, University of California at Berkeley, 1957.

91. Aranda. P: Alice Springs. G: 24°15'S, 133°30'E. T: 1896.

Murdock, G. P. Our Primitive Contemporaries, pp. 20–47. New York, 1934.

*Spencer, B., and F. J. Gillen. The Arunta. 2 vols. London, 1927.

Strehlow, C. Die Aranda und Loritja Stämme. Frankfurt am Main, 1907–11.

92. Orokaiva. P: Aiga subtribe. G: 8°30'S, 148°E. T: 1925.

Reay, M. Social Control amongst the Orokaiva. Oceania 24: 110–118. 1953.

*Williams, F. E. Orokaiva Magic. London, 1928.

*————. Orokaiva Society. London, 1930.

94. Kapauku. P: village of Botukebo. G: 4°S, 136°E. T: 1955.

*Pospisil, L. Kapauku Papuans and Their Law. Yale University Publications in Anthropology 54: 1–296. 1958.

————. Kapauku Papuans and Their Kinship Organization. Oceania 30: 188–205. 1960.

*———. Kapauku Papuan Economy. Yale University Publications in Anthropology 67: 1–502. 1963.

*———. The Kapauku Papuans of West New Guinea. New York, 1963.

95a. Wogeo. P: Wonevaro district. G: 3°S, 144°E. T: 1930.

*Hogbin, H. I. Sorcery and Administration. Oceania 6: 1–32. 1935.

*———. Native Culture in Wogeo. Oceania 6: 308–337. 1935.

———. Social Reaction to Crime. Journal of the Royal Anthropological Institute 68: 223–262. 1938.

———. Tillage and Collection: A New Guinea Economy. Oceania 9: 127–151, 286–325. 1938.

———. A New Guinea Infancy. Oceania 13: 285–309. 1943.

———. A New Guinea Childhood. Oceania 16: 275–296. 1946.

———. Sorcery and Succession in Wogeo. Oceania 23: 133–136. 1953.

96. Manus. P: village of Peri. G: 2°10′S, 147°10′E. T: 1929.

*Fortune, R. F. Manus Religion. Memoirs of the American Philosophical Society 3: 1–391. 1935.

*Mead, M. Growing Up in New Guinea. New York, 1930.

———. Kinship in the Admiralty Islands. Anthropological Papers, American Museum of Natural History 34: 180–358. 1934.

———. The Manus of the Admiralty Islands. Cooperation and Competition among Primitive Peoples, ed. M. Mead, pp. 200–239. New York, 1937.

98. Trobrianders. P: Kiriwina island. G: 8°38′S, 151°4′E. T: 1914.

*Malinowski, B. Argonauts of the Western Pacific. London, 1922.

*———. Crime and Custom in Savage Society. London, 1926.

———. The Sexual Life of Savages. 2 vols. New York, 1929.

*———. Coral Gardens and Their Magic. 2 vols. New York, 1935.

99. Siuai. P: northeastern group. G: 7°S, 155°20′E. T: 1939.

*Oliver, D. L. Studies in the Anthropology of Bougainville. Papers, Peabody Museum, Harvard University, vol. 29, nos. 1–4. 1949.

*———. A Solomon Island Society. Cambridge, 1955.

100. Tikopia. P: district of Ravenga. G: 12°30′S, 168°30′E. T: 1930.

*Firth, R. We the Tikopia. London, 1936.

*———. A Primitive Polynesian Economy. London, 1939.

*———. Work of the Gods. London School of Economics Monographs on Social Anthropology, vols. 1–2. 1940.

102. Fijians. P: island of Mbau. G: 18°S, 178°35′E. T: 1840.

Deane, W. Fijian Society. London, 1921.

*Spencer, D. M. Disease, Religion and Society in the Fiji Islands. Monographs of the American Ethnological Society 2: 1–82. 1941.

*Thomson, B. The Fijians. London, 1908.

Waterhouse, J. The King and People of Fiji. London, 1866.

*Williams, T. Fiji and the Fijians. Rev. ed. London, 1884.

103. Ajie. P: Neje chiefdom. G: 21°20′S, 165°40′E. T: 1845.

†Barrau, J. L'agriculture vivrière autochtone. Nouméa, 1956.

Guiart, J. L'organisation sociale et coutumière de la population autochtone. Nouméa, 1956.

*Leenhardt, M. Notes d'ethnologie néo-calédonie. Travaux et Mémoires de l'Institut d'Ethnologie 8: 1–340. 1930.

———. Gens de la Grande Terre, Nouvelle Calédonie. Paris, 1937.

105. Marquesans. P: southwest Nuku Hiva. G: 8°55′S, 140°10′W. T: 1800.

Handy, E. S. C. The Native Culture in the Marquesas. Bulletin of the Bernice P. Bishop Museum 9: 1–358. 1923.

†Lisiansky, R. Voyage Round the World in the Years 1803–06. London, 1814.

Miranda, P. Marquesan Social Structure. Ethnohistory 11: 301–379. 1964.

†Porter, D. A Voyage in the South Seas in the Years 1812–14. London, 1823.

Tautain. Sur l'anthropophagie et les sacrifices humains aux Iles Marquises. L'Anthropologie, 7: 542–552. 1896.

106. Samoans. P: western Upolu. G: 13°50′S, 172°W. T: 1829.

Grattan, F. J. H. An Introduction to Samoan Custom. Apia, 1948.

Krämer, A. Die Samoa-Inseln. 2 vols. Stuttgart, 1901–02.

*Stair, J. B. Old Samoa. London, 1897.

*Turner, G. Samoa. London, 1884.

108. Marshallese. P: Jaluit atoll. G: 6°N, 169°15′E. T: 1900.

*Erdland, P. A. Die Marshall-Insulaner. Münster, 1914.

*Krämer, A., and H. Nevermann. Ralik-Ratak. Ergebnisse der Südsee-Expedition 1908–1910, ed. G. Thilenius 15: 1–304. Hamburg, 1938.

Senfft, A. Die Marshall-Insulaner. Rechtsverhältnisse von eingeborenen Völker, ed. S. R. Steinmetz, pp. 425–455. Berlin, 1903.

109. Trukese. P: island of Romonum. G: 7°24′N, 151°40′E. T: 1947.

*Bollig, L. Die Bewohner der Truk-Inseln. Anthropos Ethnologische Bibliothek, vol. 3. Münster, 1927.

*Gladwin, T., and S. B. Sarason. Truk: Man in Paradise. Viking Fund Publications in Anthropology 20: 1–655. 1953.

*Goodenough, W. H. Property, Kin and Community on Truk. Yale University Publications in Anthropology 46: 1–192. 1949.

†LeBar, F. M. The Material Culture of Truk. Yale University Publications in Anthropology 68: 1–185. 1964.

111. Palauans. P: island of Koror. G: 7°N, 134°30′E. T: 1873.

*Keate, G. An Account of the Pelew Islands. London, 1788.

*Krämer, A. Palau. Ergebnisse der Südsee-Expedition 1908–1910, ed. G. Thilenius. 5 vols. Hamburg, 1929.

*Kubary, J. S. Die Palau-Inseln in der Südsee. Journal des Museum Godeffroy 1: 177–238. Hamburg, 1873.

Semper, K. Die Palau-Inseln im Stillen Ozean. Leipzig, 1873.

112. Ifugao. P: Kiangan group. G: 16°50′N, 121°10′E. T: 1910.

*Barton, R. F. Ifugao Law. University of California Publications in American Archaeology and Ethnology 15: 1–186. 1919.

———. Ifugao Economics. University of California Publications in American Archaeology and Ethnology 15: 385–466. 1922.

———. Philippine Pagans. London, 1938.

*———. The Religion of the Ifugaos. Memoirs of the American Anthropological Association 65: 1–219. 1946.

113. Atayal. G: 24°20′N, 120°35′E. T: 1930.

Mabuchi, T. The Aboriginal Peoples of Formosa. Viking Fund Publications in Anthropology 29: 127–140. 1960.

*Okada, Y. The Social Structure of the Aatayal Tribe (manuscript translated from Essays presented to Teizo Toda, pp. 393–433). Tokyo, 1949.

Ruey Yih-fu. Ethnographical Investigations of Some Aspects of the Atayal. Bulletin, Department of Archaeology and Anthropology, National Taiwan University 5: 113–127. 1955.

115. Manchu. P: Aigun district. G: 50°N, 125°30′E. T: 1915.

*Shirokogoroff, S. M. Social Organization of the Manchus. Royal Asiatic Society, North China Branch, Extra Volume 3. Shanghai, 1924.

117. Japanese. P: southern Okayama prefecture. G: 34°40′N, 133°48′E. T: 1950.

*Beardsley, R. K., J. W. Hall, and R. E. Ward. Village Japan. Ann Arbor, 1956.

†DeVos, G. Social Values and Personal Attitudes in Primary Human Relations in Niiike. University of Michigan Center for Japanese Studies, Occasional Papers, Ann Arbor, 1965.

*Norbeck, E. Takashima. Salt Lake City, 1954.

Smith, R. S., and J. B. Cornell. Two Japanese Villages. Ann Arbor, 1956.

118. Ainu. P: Saru basin. G: 42°50′N, 143°E. T: 1880.

*Batchelor, J. Ainu Life and Lore. Tokyo, 1927.

*Hilger, M. I. Together with the Ainu. Norman, 1971.

*Munro, N. G. Ainu Creed and Cult, ed. B. Z. Seligman. New York, 1962.

†Sugiura, S., and H. Befu. Kinship Organization of the Saru Ainu. Ethnology 1: 287–298. 1962.

Watanabe, H. The Ainu. Journal of the Faculty of Science, University of Tokyo, Anthropology 2: vi, 1–164. 1964.

120. Yukaghir. P: on upper Kolyma River. G: 65°N, 155°E. T: 1850.

*Jochelson, W. The Yukaghir and Yukaghirized Tungus. Memoirs of the American Museum of Natural History 13: 1–469. 1926.

121. Chukchee. P: Reindeer division. G: 67°N, 180°E. T: 1900.

*Bogoras, W. The Chukchee. Memoirs of the American Museum of Natural History 11: 1–703. 1904–09.

Sverdrup, H. U. Hos tendrafolket. Oslo, 1938.

122. Ingalik. P: village of Shageluk. G: 62°30'N, 159°30'W. T: 1885.

Osgood, C. Ingalik Material Culture. Yale University Publications in Anthropology 22: 1–500. 1940.

*———. Ingalik Social Culture. Yale University Publications in Anthropology 55: 1–289. 1958.

*———. Ingalik Mental Culture. Yale University Publications in Anthropology 56: 1–195. 1959.

123. Aleut. P: Unalaska division. G: 55°N, 164°W. T: 1778.

Bank, T. P. Health and Medical Lore of the Aleuts. Papers of the Michigan Academy of Science, Arts, and Letters 38: 415–431. 1953.

Cook, J. A Voyage to the Pacific Ocean. London, 1785.

*Lantis, M. Ethnohistory in Southwestern Alaska and the Southern Yukon. Lexington, 1970.

Sarytschev, G. An Account of a Voyage of Discovery. 2 vols. London, 1806.

*Veniaminov, I. E. P. Zapiski ob ostrovakh unalashkinskago otdela. St. Petersburg, 1840.

124. Copper Eskimo. P: mainland division. G: 68°N, 113°W. T: 1915.

*Jenness, D. The Life of the Copper Eskimos. Report of the Canadian Arctic Expedition, 1913–18, 12: 5–227. 1922.

*———. People of the Twilight. New York, 1928.

Rasmussen, K. Intellectual Culture of the Copper Eskimos. Report of the Fifth Thule Expedition 9: 1–350. 1932.

Stefansson, V. The Stefansson-Anderson Arctic Expedition. Anthropological Papers, American Museum of Natural History 14: i, 1–395. 1914.

126. Micmac. P: mainland division. G: 45°N, 63°W. T: 1650.

Denys, N. The Description and Natural History of the Coasts of North America. Publications of the Champlain Society 2: 399–452, 572–606. 1908.

Johnson, F. Notes on Micmac Shamanism. Primitive Man 16: 53–80. 1943.

*Le Clercq, C. New Relation of Gaspesia. Publications of the Champlain Society 5: 1–452. 1910.

127. Saulteaux. P: Berens River band. G: 52°N, 96°W. T: 1930.

*Hallowell, A. I. Fear and Anxiety as Cultural and Individual Variables in a Primitive Society. Journal of Social Psychology 9: 25–47. 1938.

*———. Sin, Sex and Sickness in Saulteaux Belief. British Journal of Medical Psychology 18: 191–197. 1939.

*———. Aggression in Saulteaux Society. Psychiatry 3: 395–407. 1940.

*———. The Social Function of Anxiety in a Primitive Society. American Sociological Review 6: 869–881. 1941.

*———. The Role of Conjuring in Saulteaux Society. Publications, Philadelphia Anthropological Society 2: 1–96. 1942.

*———. Culture and Experience. Philadelphia, 1955.

*———. Ojibwa World View and Disease. Man's Image in Medicine and Anthropology, ed. I. Goldstone, pp. 258–315. New York, 1963.

128. Slave. P: Lynx Point band. G: 62°N, 122°W. T: 1940.

Helm, J. The Lynx Point People. Bulletin, National Museum of Canada 176: 1–193. 1961.

*Honigmann, J. Ethnography and Acculturation of the Fort Nelson Slave. Yale University Publications in Anthropology: 33: 1–169. 1946.

*MacNeish, June Helm. Leadership among the Northeastern Athapascans. Anthropologica 2: 131–163. 1960.

*Mason, J. A. Notes on the Indians of the Great Slave Lake Area. Yale University Publications in Anthropology 34: 1–46. 1946.

129. Kaska. P: along the upper Liard River. G: 60°N, 131°W. T: 1900.

*Honigmann, J. Culture and Ethos of Kaska Society. Yale University Publications in Anthropology 40: 1–368. 1949.

*———. The Kaska Indians. Yale University Publications in Anthropology 51: 1–163. 1954.

Teit, J. A. Field Notes on the Tahltan and Kaska Indians. Anthropologica 3: 39–171. 1956.

131. Haida. P: village of Masset. G: 54°N, 132°30′W. T: 1875.

*Murdock, G. P. Our Primitive Contemporaries, pp. 221–263. New York, 1934.

———. Kinship and Social Behavior among the Haida. American Anthropologist 36: 355–385. 1934.

†———. Rank and Potlatch among the Haida. Yale University Publications in Anthropology 13: 1–20. 1936.

†Niblack, A. P. The Coastal Indians of Southern Alaska and Northern British Columbia. Annual Reports, United States National Museum, 1888, pp. 225–386.

*Swanton, J. R. Contributions to the Ethnology of the Haida. Memoirs of the American Museum of Natural History 8: 1–300. 1909.

132. Bellacoola. G: 52°20′N, 126°30′W. T: 1880.
*Boas, F. The Bilqula. Report, British Association for the Advancement of Science 61: 408–424. 1891.
†Drucker, P. Northwest Coast. Anthropological Records 9: 157–294. 1950.
*McIlwraith, T. F. The Bella Coola Indians. 2 vols. Toronto, 1948.
Smith, H. I. Sympathetic Magic and Witchcraft among the Bellacoola. American Anthropologist 27: 116–121. 1964.

133. Twana. G: 47°25′N, 123°15′W. T: 1860.
*Eells, M. Twana Indians of the Skokomish Reservation. Bulletin, United States Geological and Geographical Survey of the Territories 3: 57–114. 1877.
*Elmendorf, W. W. The Structure of Twana Culture. Washington State University Research Studies Monographic Supplement 2: 1–576. 1960.

134. Yurok. P: village of Tsurai. G: 41°30′N, 124°W. T: 1850.
*Erikson, E. H. Observations on the Yurok. University of California Publications in American Archaeology and Ethnology 25: 257–302. 1943.
†Heizer, R. F., and J. E. Mills. The Four Ages of Tsurai. Berkeley, 1952.
*Kroeber, A. L. Handbook of the Indians of California. Bulletin, Bureau of American Ethnology 78: 1–97. 1925.
Waterman, T. T., and A. L. Kroeber. Yurok Marriages. University of California Publications in American Archaeology and Ethnology 35: 1–14. 1934.

135. Eastern Pomo. P: village of Cigon. G: 39°N, 123°W. T: 1850.
†Barrett, S. A. Material Aspects of Pomo Culture. Bulletin, Public Museum of the City of Milwaukee 20: 1–508. 1952.
*Freeland, L. S. Pomo Doctors and Poisoners. University of California Publications in American Archaeology and Ethnology 20: 57–73. 1923.
Gifford, E. W. Clear Lake Pomo Society. University of California Publications in American Archaeology and Ethnology 18: 287–390. 1926.
Gifford, E. W., and A. L. Kroeber. Pomo. University of California Publications in American Archaeology and Ethnology 37: 117–254. 1937.
*Loeb, E. M. Pomo Folkways. University of California Publications in American Archaeology and Ethnology 19: 149–405. 1926.

137. Paiute. P: Wadadika of Harney Valley. G: 43°30′N, 119°W. T: 1870.
Stewart, O. C. Northern Paiute Bands. Anthropological Records 2: 127–149. 1937.
*——. Northern Paiute. Anthropological Records 4: 361–446. 1941.

*Whiting, B. B. Paiute Sorcery. Viking Fund Publications in Anthropology 15: 1–110. 1950.

138. Klamath. G: 42°40′N, 121°50′W. T: 1860.

*Gatschet, A. S. The Klamath Indians of Southwestern Oregon. Contributions to North American Ethnology 2. 2 vols. 1890.

Pearsall, M. Klamath Childhood and Education. Anthropological Records 9: 339–351. 1950.

*Spier, L. Klamath Ethnography. University of California Publications in American Archaeology and Ethnology 30: 1–338. 1930.

Stern, T. The Klamath Tribe. Seattle, 1965.

Voegelin, E. W. Northeast California. Anthropological Records 7: 47–251. 1942.

139. Kutenai. P: lower or eastern branch. G: 49°N, 116°40′W. T: 1890.

Boas, F. Kutenai Tales. Bulletin, Bureau of American Ethnology 59: 1–387. 1918.

Chamberlain, A. F. Report on the Kootenay Indians. Report, British Association for the Advancement of Science 4: 549–617. 1892.

*Ray, V. F. Plateau. Anthropological Records 8: 99–262. 1942.

*Turney-High, H. H. Ethnography of the Kutenai. Memoirs of the American Anthropological Association 56: 1–202. 1941.

141a. Crow. G: 45°N, 109°W. T: 1870.

Lowie, R. H. Social Life of the Crow Indians. Anthropological Papers, American Museum of Natural History 9: 179–248. 1912.

———. The Material Culture of the Crow Indians. Anthropological Papers, American Museum of Natural History 21: 201–270. 1922.

*———. The Religion of the Crow Indians. Anthropological Papers, American Museum of Natural History 25: 309–444. 1922.

*———. The Crow Indians. New York, 1935.

142. Pawnee. P: Skidi band. 42°N, 100°W. T: 1867.

Dorsey, G. A. Traditions of the Skidi Pawnee. Memoirs of the American Folk-Lore Society 8: 1–366. 1904.

Dorsey, G. A., and J. R. Murie. Notes on Skidi Pawnee Society. Field Museum of Natural History Anthropological Series 27: 65–119. 1940.

†Lounsbury, F. G. A Semantic Analysis of the Pawnee Kinship Usage. Language 32: 158–194. 1956.

*Weltfish, G. The Lost Universe. New York, 1965.

143. Omaha. G: 41°25′N, 96°30′W. T: 1860.

Dorsey, J. O. Omaha Sociology. Annual Report, Bureau of American Ethnology 3: 205–320. 1884.

Appendix 117

*Fletcher, A. C., and F. LaFlesche. The Omaha Tribe. Annual Report, Bureau of American Ethnology 27: 17–672. 1911.

Fortune, R. F. Omaha Secret Societies. Columbia University Contributions to Anthropology 14: 1–193. 1932.

Mead, M. The Changing Culture of an Indian Tribe. Columbia University Contributions to Anthropology 15: 1–313. 1932.

144. Huron. P: Attignawantan and Attigneenongnahac. G: 44°30′N, 79°W. T: 1634.

*Kinietz, W. V. The Indians of the Western Great Lakes. Occasional Contributions from the Museum of Anthropology, University of Michigan 10: 1–160. 1940.

*Tooker, E. An Ethnography of the Huron Indians, 1615–1649. Bulletin, Bureau of American Ethnology 190: 1–183. 1964.

*Trigger, B. C. The Huron. New York, 1969.

147. Comanche. G: 34°N, 102°W. T: 1870.

†Gladwin, T. Comanche Kin Behavior. American Anthropologist 50: 73–94. 1948.

*Hoebel, E. A. The Political Organization and Law-Ways of the Comanche Indians. Memoirs of the American Anthropological Association 54: 1–149. 1940.

*Wallace, E., and E. A. Hoebel. The Comanches. Norman, 1948.

148. Chiricahua Apache. P: Central band. G: 32°N, 109°30′W. T: 1870.

Gifford, E. W. Apache-Pueblo. Anthropological Records 4: 1–207. 1940.

*Opler, M. E. Some Points of Comparison and Contrast between the Treatment of Functional Disorders by Apache Shamans and Modern Psychiatric Practice. American Journal of Psychiatry 92: 1371–1387. 1936.

———. An Outline of Chiricahua Apache Social Organization. Social Organization of North American Tribes, ed. F. Eggan, pp. 173–239. Chicago, 1937.

*———. An Apache Life-Way. Chicago, 1941.

149. Zuni. G: 35°40′N, 108°45′W. T: 1880.

*Bunzel, R. Introduction to Zuni Ceremonialism. Annual Report, Bureau of American Ethnology 47: 467–544. 1964.

Eggan, F. Social Organization of the Western Pueblos. Chicago, 1950.

*Leighton, D. C., and J. Adair. People of the Middle Place. New Haven, 1966.

Roberts, J. M. Zuni Daily Life. New Haven, 1965.

Smith, W., and J. M. Roberts. Zuni Law. Papers of the Peabody Museum, Harvard University 43: 1–185. 1954.

*Stevenson, M. C. The Zuni Indians. Annual Report, Bureau of American Ethnology 23: 13–608. 1904.

150. Havasupai. G: 35°50′N, 112°W. T: 1918.

Cushing, F. H. The Nation of the Willows. Atlantic Monthly 50: 362–374, 541–559. 1882.

Smithson, C. L. The Havasupai Woman. University of Utah Anthropological Papers 38: 1–170. 1950.

*Spier, L. Havasupai Ethnography. Anthropological Papers, American Museum of Natural History 29: 83–392. 1928.

153. Aztec. P: city and environs of Tenochtitlan. G: 19°N, 99°10′W. T: 1520.

*Sahagun, B. de. Florentine Codex, trans. A. J. O. Anderson and C. F. Dibble. Monographs of the School of American Research 14, pts. 2, 3, 4, 8, 13, 14. Santa Fe, 1950–57.

*Soustelle, J. Daily Life of the Aztecs. New York, 1961.

Thompson, J. R. Mexico before Cortez. New York, 1933.

Vaillant, G. C. Aztecs of Mexico. New York, 1941.

154. Popoluca. P: town and environs of Soteapan. G: 18°15′N, 94°50′W. T: 1940.

*Foster, G. M. Notes on the Popoluca of Veracruz. Publicaciones del Instituto Panamericano de Geografia e Historia 51: 1–41. 1940.

———. A Primitive Mexican Economy. Monographs of the American Ethnological Society 5: 1–115. 1940.

*———. Sierra Popoluca Folklore and Beliefs. University of California Publications in American Archaeology and Ethnology 42: 177–250. 1945. 1945.

155. Quiche. P: town of Chichicastenango. G: 15°N, 91°W. T: 1930.

*Bunzel, R. Chichicastenango. Publications of the American Ethnological Society 22: 1–438. 1952.

*Schultze-Jena, L. Indiana I: Leben, Glaube und Sprache der Quiché von Guatemala. Jena, 1933.

156. Miskito. P: village near Cape Gracias a Dios. G: 15°N, 83°W. T: 1921.

*Conzemius, E. Ethnographic Survey of the Miskito and Sumu Indians. Bulletin, Bureau of American Ethnology 106: 1–191. 1932.

†Helms, M. W. The Cultural Ecology of a Colonial Tribe. Ethnology 8: 76–84. 1969.

*———. Asang. Gainesville, 1971.

Pijoan, M. The Health and Customs of the Miskito Indians. Mexico: Instituto Indigena Interamericano, 1946.

159. Cuna. P: San Blas islands. G: 9°15′N, 78°30′W. T: 1927.

†Krieger, H. W. Material Culture of the People of Southeastern Panama.

Bulletin, United States National Museum 134: 1–133. 1926.

*Nordenskiöld, E. An Historical and Ethnological Survey of the Cuna Indians. Comparative Ethnological Studies 10: 1–686. Göteborg, 1938.

*Stout, D. C. San Blas Acculturation. Viking Fund Publications in Anthropology 9: 1–124. 1947.

*Wafer, L. A New Voyage and Description of the Isthmus of America, ed. L. E. E. Joyce. Hakluyt Society, ser. 2, vol. 73. Oxford, 1934.

159. Goajiro. G: 12°N, 71°45'W. T: 1947.

Bolinder, G. Indians on Horseback. London, 1957.

*Gutierrez de Pineda, V. Organización social en la Guajira. Revista del Instituto Etnológico Nacional 3: ii, 1–255. Bogotá, 1948.

*Pineda Giraldo, R. Aspectos de la magia en la Guajira. Revista del Instituto Etnológico Nacional 3: i, 1–164. Bogotá, 1950.

Simons, F. A. A. An Exploration of the Goajira Peninsula. Proceedings of the Royal Geographical Society, n.s., 7: 781–796. 1885.

Wilbert, J. Literatura oral y creencias de los Indios Goajiro. Caracas, 1962.

160. Haitians. P: Mirebalais. G: 18°50'N, 72°10'W. T: 1935.

†Bastien, R. La familia haitiana. Mexico, 1951.

*Herskovits, M. J. Life in a Haitian Valley. New York, 1937.

Leyburn, J. G. The Haitian People. New Haven, 1941.

*Métraux, A. Haiti Black Peasants and Their Religion. Neuchâtel, 1960.

162. Warrau. P: Orinoco delta. G: 9°10'N, 62°W. 1935.

Suárez, M. M. Los Warao. Caracas, 1968.

*Turrado Moreno, A. Etnographia de los Indios Guaranos. Caracas, 1945.

*Wilbert, J. Die soziale und politische Organisation der Warrau. Kölner Zeitschrift für Soziologie und Sozialpsychologie, n.s., 10: 272–291. 1958.

*———. Warao Oral Literature. Caracas, 1964.

165. Saramacca. P: on upper Suriname River. G: 3°30'N, 55°45'W. T: 1932.

†Neumann, P. Wirtschaft und materielle Kultur der Buschneger Surinames. Abhandlungen und Berichte des staatlichen Museum für Völkerkunde zu Dresden 26: 1–181. 1967.

*Price, R. Saramaka Social Structure. Caribbean Monograph Series 12: 1–181. 1975.

166. Mundurucu. P: village of Cabrua. G: 7°S, 57°W. T: 1950.

†Murphy, R. F. Matrilocality and Patrilinearity in Mundurucú Society. American Anthropologist 58: 414–434. 1956.

*———. Mundurucú Religion. University of California Publications in American Anthropological Association 68: 1–250. 1948.

*———. Headhunter's Heritage. Berkeley, 1960.

167. Cubeo. P: village on the Caduiari River. G: 1°25'S, 70°30'W. T: 1939.

*Goldman, I. The Cubeo Indians. Illinois Studies in Anthropology 2: 1–305. 1963.

169. Jivaro. G: 3°S, 78°W. T: 1920.

*Harner, M. J. Machetes, Shotguns and Society. Ph.D. dissertation, University of California at Berkeley, 1960.

*Karsten, R. The Head-Hunters of Western Amazonas. Societas Scientiarum Fennica, Commentationes Humanarum Litterarum 7: 1–588. 1935.

Rivet, P. Les Indiens Jibáros. L'Anthropologie 18: 333–368, 583–618; 19: 68–87, 235–259. 1907–08.

Stirling, M. W. Historical and Ethnographic Material on the Jivaro Indians. Bulletin, Bureau of American Ethnology 117: 1–148. 1938.

170. Amahuaca. P: on upper Inuya River. G: 10°20'S, 72°15'W. T: 1960.

Carneiro, R. L. The Amahuaca Indians. Explorers Journal 40: iv, 28–37. 1962.

*———. The Amahuaca and the Spirit World. Ethnology 3: 6–11. 1964.

*Huxley, M., and C. Capa. Farewell to Eden. New York, 1964

Tessmann, G. Die Indianer Nordost-Perus. Hamburg, 1930.

171. Inca. P: city and environs of Cuzco. G: 13°30'S, 72°W. T: 1530.

*Mason, J. A. The Ancient Civilizations of Peru. London, 1957.

Means, P. A. Ancient Civilizations of the Andes. New York, 1931.

Murdock, G. P. Our Primitive Contemporaries, pp. 403–450. New York, 1934.

*Rowe, J. H. Inca Culture at the Time of the Conquest. Bulletin, Bureau of American Ethnology 143: ii, 183–330. 1946.

172. Aymara. P: an *ayllu* near Chucuito. G: 16°S, 70°W. T: 1940.

LaBarre, W. The Aymara Indians of the Lake Titicaca Plateau. Memoirs, American Anthropological Association 68: 1–250. 1948.

*Tschopik, H., Jr. The Aymara. Bulletin, Bureau of American Ethnology 143: ii, 501–573. 1946.

*———. The Aymara of Chucuito. Anthropological Papers, American Museum of Natural History 44: 137–308. 1948.

173. Siriono. P: near the Rio Blanco. G: 14°30'S, 63°30'W. T: 1942.

*Holmberg, A. R. Nomads of the Long Bow. Publications of the Institute of Social Anthropology, Smithsonian Institution 10: 1–104. 1950.

175a. Bororo. P: village of Kejara. G: 15°45'S, 54°45'W. T: 1935.

Cook, W. A. Through the Wildernesses of Brazil. New York, 1909.

Fric, V. A., and P. Radin. Contributions to the Study of the Bororo Indians. Journal of the Royal Anthropological Institute 36: 382–406. 1906.

Lévi-Strauss, C. Contribution à l'étude de l'organisation sociale des Indiens

Appendix

Bororo. Journal de la Société des Américanistes 28: 269–304. 1936.

*Lowie, R. H. The Bororo. Bulletin, Bureau of American Ethnology 143: i, 419–434. 1953.

*Steinen, K. von den. Unter den Naturvölkern Zentral-Brasiliens. Berlin, 1894.

176. Timbira. P: Ramcocamecra or Canella subtribe. G: 6°30′S, 45°30′W. T: 1915.

Crocker, W. H. The Canela since Nimuendaju. Anthropological Quarterly 23: 69–84. 1961.

Kissenberth, W. Bei den Canella-Indianern in Zentral Maranhas. Baessler-Archiv 2: 45–54. 1912.

*Nimuendajú, C. The Eastern Timbira. University of California Publications in American Archaeology and Ethnology 41: 1–357. 1946.

Snethlage, E. H. Unter nordostbrasilianischen Indianern. Zeitschrift für Ethnologie 62: 111–205. 1930.

177. Tupinamba. P: village near Rio de Janeiro. G: 22°50′S, 43°15′W. T: 1550.

Léry, J. de. Histoire d'un voyage faict en la terre du Brésil. Paris, 1880.

*Métraux, A. The Tupinamba. Bulletin, Bureau of American Ethnology 143: iii, 95–133. 1948.

Soares de Souza, G. Tratato descriptivo do Brasil em 1587. Revista do Instituto Histórico e Geográphico do Brazil 14: 1–423. 1851.

Staden, H. The True Story of His Captivity, ed. M. Lotts. London, 1928.

*Thevet, A. Les singularitez de la France antarctique, ed. P. Gaffarel. Paris, 1878.

Yves d'Evreux. Voyage dans le nord Brésil, ed. F. Denis. Leipzig and Paris, 1864.

179a. Caraja. P: west bank of Araguaya River. G: 12°40′S, 51°E. T: 1908.

†Dietschy, H. Geburtshütte und "Männerkindbett" bei den Karajá. Verhandlungen der Naturforschenden Gesellschaft zu Basel 68: 114–132. 1956.

*Ehrenreich, P. Beiträge zur Völkerkunde Brasiliens. Veröffentlichungen aus dem Königlichen Museum für Völkerkunde 2: 1–80. Leipzig, 1891.

*Krause, F. In den Wildnissen Brasiliens. Leipzig, 1911.

*Lipkind, W. The Carajá. Bulletin, Bureau of American Ethnology 143: iii, 179–191. 1948.

180. Aweikoma. P: Duque de Caxias Reservation. G: 28°S, 50°W. T: 1932.

*Henry, J. Jungle People. New York, 1941.

Métraux, A. The Caingang. Bulletin, Bureau of American Ethnology 143: i, 445–475. 1946.

182. Lengua. G: 23°30'S, 58°30'W. T: 1889.

Baldus, H. Indianerstudien im nordöstlichen Chaco. Forschungen zur Völkerpsychologie und Soziologie 11: 1–239. 1931.

*Grubb, W. B. An Unknown People in an Unknown Land. London, 1911.

Hawtrey, S. H. C. The Lengua Indians of the Paraguayan Chaco. Journal of the Royal Anthropological Institute 31: 280–299. 1901.

184. Mapuche. P: vicinity of Temuco. G: 38°30'S, 72°35'W. T: 1950.

Faron, L. C. Mapuche Social Structure. Illinois Studies in Anthropology 1: 1–247. 1961.

*———. Hawks of the Sun. Pittsburgh, 1964.

*———. The Mapuche Indians of Chile. New York, 1968.

†Hilger, M. I. Araucanian Child Life and Its Cultural Background. Smithsonian Miscellaneous Collections 133: 1–495. 1957.

*Titiev, M. Araucanian Culture in Transition. Occasional Contributions from the Museum of Anthropology, University of Michigan 15: 1–164. 1951.

185. Tehuelche. G: 45°S, 68°W. T: 1870.

†Bourne, B. F. The Captive in Patagonia. Boston, 1874.

Cooper, J. M. The Patagonian and Pampean Hunters. Bulletin, Bureau of of American Ethnology 143: i, 127–268. 1946.

*Musters, G. C. At Home with the Patagonians. London, 1874.

*Viedma, A. de. Descripción de la costa meridional del sur. Collección de obras y documentos relativos a la historia antigua y modern de la provincias del Rio de la Plata, ed. P. de Angelis 6: 63–81. Buenos Aires, 1837.

186. Yahgan. G: 55°30'S, 70°W. T: 1865.

Cooper, J. M. An Analytical and Critical Bibliography of the Tribes of Tierra del Fuego. Bulletin, Bureau of American Ethnology 63: 1–243. 1917.

*———. The Yahgan. Bulletin, Bureau of American Ethnology 143: i, 81–106. 1946.

*Gusinde, M. Die Feuerland-Indianer 2: Yamana. Mödling bei Wien, 1937.

Index

123